Unlock Your Macro Type

Unlock Your
MACRO TYPE

Identify Your True Body Type

Understand Your Carb Tolerance

Accelerate Fat Loss

CHRISTINE HRONEC, M.S.

Founder, Gauge Girl Training

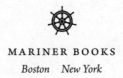

MARINER BOOKS

Boston   New York

marinerbooks.com

Library of Congress Cataloging-in-Publication Data has been applied for.
ISBN 978-0-358-576624

Printed in the United States of America
1 2022

Contents

Introduction

L ike many women, I struggled with fat loss. As a teenager in the '90s, I wanted to look like Kate Moss, but no matter what I did, my body would not and could not transform into a super-thin frame. I ran cross-country, I rollerbladed, I did workout videos ranging from Denise Austin to Tae Bo every day, but it never seemed to make any difference.

I didn't know what to do. I felt like a failure. I felt like the only way I could reach my goal was to have a superhuman amount of willpower that I would never possess. (Sound familiar?) Because of this, I struggled with my body image for a long time. Why was it that I could crush all my academic and career goals, but when it came to my physique, I couldn't do anything to accomplish what I wanted? I tried fasting, Atkins, juicing, vegetarianism, veganism, the cabbage soup diet, the Special K diet, diet pills, you name it. If there was a commercialized solution to weight loss in the '90s and early 2000s, I promise you, I tried it.

When these plans didn't work, I convinced myself that I wasn't working hard enough. I thought if I could just do more cardio, I would have visible abs. So, guess what? I became a marathon runner. For two years, I ran 40 to 50 miles a week . . . and I didn't lose any weight! My runner's body didn't have the lean, athletic look I was after. To add insult to injury, I felt hungry all the time. This pissed me off. I wasn't afraid of hard work, but what I was doing wasn't getting results. I was sick and tired of feeling powerless.

As I struggled with my fitness goals, my career in chemical engineering and food science was taking off. My work led me to the dietary supplement industry, where I cofounded a dietary supplement manufacturing company and built a production plant. As part of my job, I formulated and developed thousands of products for various businesses. I lived between the lab, the plant, and my Excel spreadsheets. My lab notebooks documented every variable of every experiment I ran for an entire decade. I had a Six Sigma Green Belt from DuPont and was an expert at statistical data analysis. As a biochemical engineer, I applied science-based, data-driven principles to solving problems every day, which raised the question: *Why on earth was I not doing this for my body?*

It was inevitable that these two passions of my life — science and wellness — would intersect.

After trying every diet under the sun and feeling frustrated for years, I applied my knowledge of science and experimental design to my own body and prepared a protocol for myself consisting of weight training, cardio, and macros-based nutrition (eating a specific breakdown of protein, fat, and carbohydrates). In other words, I determined how to adjust what I ate — how I fueled my body — in a measurable way that would shift my body composition to consuming more protein and less fat. Most plans measure what you eat by one metric only, calorie count, but don't take into account the breakdown of those calories, which — as you'll discover throughout this book — can make all of the difference.

Like many of you, I've been there, done that when it comes to reducing calories and never got my desired results. Once I applied science to my diet — monitoring the protein, carb, and fat composition of my calories — it completely changed the game, and my life has never been the same. Soon after, I took my newfound six-pack abs and won second place in my first fitness competition. I was hooked.

Ten years ago, following my sudden breakthrough, someone sent me a question through social media: "How did you transform your physique with such success?" I made a video responding to it. And then another. And another. Once I started making educational YouTube videos and watched as the videos gained in popularity, I began to realize just how many people are confused about nutrition. In the YouTube comments, in emails, on the street, people started asking me for weight-loss programs and coaching. Soon a few requests became a few hundred, until an overwhelming number of people were asking me to help them understand where they were going wrong and show them the way to a healthier physique. I took on my first client as a health coach in 2013.

While I saw great success with many of my clients, it soon became clear to me that what worked for my body didn't work for everyone. That's when I began to refine my program, customizing plans to complement a person's biological profile. In the last decade, I've helped over 40,000 clients improve their health with this very process.

What I offer you in these pages is the result of a decade of health coaching. It's not a guide to what everyone should be eating and doing, but a guide to what *you* should be eating and how *you* should be working out to achieve the best body for *you*. Everyone's body responds to different foods in different ways. If you read a book about dieting in the past, and it didn't work for you, it probably ignored this simple fact. Every dieting book out there worked for the person who wrote it, but whether or not their approach will be right for you is another set of questions entirely — questions I'll be asking (and helping you answer) in this book.

In broad terms, this approach gauges the suitability of a particular diet for you based on certain bio-individual factors. These include your carb tolerance, caloric intake, and what I call your macro type — a categorization that takes your personal carb tolerance and body type into account to help customize a plan that will work best for your body. My approach demands a shift in perspective, which I encourage you to adopt: Nutrition is not a question of what to eliminate from your diet, but an understanding of what you need to consume.

This method — macro-typing — provides the most effective framework for science-based meal planning. That one question from so many years ago — "How did you transform your physique with such success?" — has grown into a movement, with over 40,000 individuals who have worked with me and found success using macro-based nutrition protocols, and 30 million YouTube viewers who have learned about the science of macronutrients. This method *works*.

The days of one-size-fits-all fat loss and meal planning are over. This book will give you a road map to navigate your nutritional needs in the way that's most appropriate for you. I've seen far too many women try diet plans built for men or who are taught that carbs are "bad," with no context as to whether or not carbs are right for *them*. In this book, you will gain a deeper understanding of how your body responds to carbohydrates and what level is suitable for your specific needs (it's likely much higher than you realize!). You will learn which nutrients you need in larger quantities and why you need them. I'll share the latest scientific research, and you'll learn how to connect the dots about how your body works and what it needs. From there, you will proceed to your plan with the confidence that you are navigating your health goals based on actual science so you can get actual results.

I recommend approaching this book with an open mind. Having tried many nutrition strategies myself, I understand that past experiences have a way of sticking around and shaping our perceptions of new ideas about nutrition. (How many times have you tried a new plan and thought, *Here I go again?* I know I felt that way before I created this program.) I challenge you to bring those past experiences along with you so you can compare and contrast those with what you learn here. This way, you'll be able to see clearly how they measure up and exactly where *they failed you.*

Some of the hard questions you'll want to ask yourself are:

- Have you been cutting out carbs with no practical reason to do so?
- Which macros have you been eating? How do your eating patterns compare to what your body needs? Which foods have you been leaving out that are preventing you from reaching your goals?
- Which macronutrients do you tend to overeat?
- How can you optimize timing your carb intake with respect to your workout?

In addition to a lot of hard-hitting yet accessible science, this book contains quizzes to help you determine your carb tolerance level, macro type, and recommended caloric intake, as well as training guidelines and meal plans, with my arsenal of handcrafted recipes to boot.

I know it's tempting, but *please* resist the urge to jump right to the quizzes and meal plans and recipes. If you go straight to these elements without knowing the science behind them, you will not be able to use them to their fullest potential, and you will be doing yourself a disservice.

For the best results, I recommend reading this book all the way through once to understand the five macro types and why they exist. Then I encourage you to take a second pass, this time focusing on the quizzes and zeroing in on your specific macro type. From there, use the book as a reference when you need a refresher on the relationship between nutrition and biochemistry or when you need a fresh, macro-appropriate recipe. (The spicy pickles are one of my favorites.) I send you off with confidence, knowing that this book has the potential to change your life for the better. This plan shines the light on the areas of your health that need attention and are *so easy* to address with proper knowledge. You only have this one body: It's yours and no one else's. It's up to you to learn how to treat it with the utmost love, care, and respect it deserves. It's time to invest energy into living your best life!

TRAINING PLANS FOR EACH MACRO TYPE

Training plans for each macro type can be accessed online. Using an Apple or Android smart phone, open the **Camera app.** Select the rear-facing camera and hold the device so that the QR code appears in the viewfinder. Your  device will recognize the QR code with a notification to take you to the web address. Exercise descriptions can be found here as well.

1

Why Macro Types?

I n the last two decades, there has been a drastic change in the way people get information on nutrition, health, and wellness. The rise of social media has transformed the landscape. We're bombarded with more information than ever. Unfortunately, most of this content is of unreliable quality and reinforces inaccurate ideals of health and body image. It's no wonder many of us are left feeling confused, overwhelmed, and with a sinking feeling that we will never truly measure up, no matter how hard we try.

Have you ever felt like something is just "off" with your ability to lose fat? Like no matter how hard you try — how many hours you log at the gym or how many calories you count — your body just refuses to budge, leaving you feeling defeated? Do you ever wonder why some individuals can eat tons of carbs and never gain a pound, yet if you eat just one carb, you seem bloated for days? Do you feel hungry for "real food" even when you are applying your best efforts to eat clean meals? Does it feel like your efforts just aren't landing you where you want to be physique-wise, and you are considering either giving up altogether or trying a more extreme approach to just get this over and done with?

If this is you, you are not alone, and you are in the right place. You may have blamed yourself for your limited success with diet plans in the past when you made drastic cuts to your caloric intake and deprived your body of key nutrients without knowing it. While extreme calorie restriction may work for the first week or so, it cannot and will not sustain results. Your body *needs* nutrients to function. Your organs, your brain, your bodily systems, your hormones, and your muscles need energy to perform. The world we live in is looking at nutrition completely backwards. Instead of looking at it through the lens of *What nutrients does my body need to thrive?* we approach it thinking, *Let me cut my calories and take this energy away from my body in the hopes that the stars will align and I will magically shrink.* The human body is far more complex than that. Fat loss is a science, not a pipe dream.

Your body needs specific nutrients in large quantities. These are known as *macronutrients* (aka macros). The three macros that your body requires are proteins, carbohydrates, and fats. If you go below a critical level of the nutrients your body requires, it can induce serious biochemical, hormonal, or metabolic imbalances. You cannot trick the body into burning body fat at a rate faster than it can, but you *can* lose weight faster and more effectively by understanding the nutrients you need, balancing your macronutrient ratios and targeting the type of nutritional approach that will be most suitable for you.

The era of one-size-fits-most nutrition plans is over. The broad spectrum between what the USDA says we need to eat in a day, what the fitness/bodybuilding community says we need, and what the "keto-Atkins-paleo-high-fat-low-carb" world says we need can be baffling.

So where do you begin? We need to start with realistic expectations about what we *can* control and what we *cannot*.

THINGS YOU CAN CONTROL

- You can reduce your overall body fat percentage.
- You can add toned muscle.
- You can control what you eat.

- You can control how much you eat.
- You can control when you eat.

THINGS YOU CANNOT CONTROL

- You cannot spot-reduce body fat.
- You cannot control where your body tends to store excess body fat.
- You cannot control how easily you can gain muscle.
- You cannot control how easily you can lose body fat.
- You cannot control how easily you can gain body fat.
- You cannot control how long it's going to take to drop true body fat.

It's essential to have realistic expectations about how long it's going to take to achieve an ideal body fat percentage, how much effort is required, and what is possible based on physical abilities, anatomy, and genetics. You can control your body fat percentage, and you can add muscle size and definition through proper nutrition. However, there are some things that impact how you look that you cannot control, such as *where* your body tends to store fat, how easily you can lose fat, how easily you can gain muscle, and how easily you can gain fat. Even an aggressive training and nutrition regimen can only have a slight impact on how long it takes to truly drop body fat. For the most part, even 100 percent adherence to a nutrition and training plan cannot accelerate this rate. One of the simplest ways to begin dialing in your protocol is to consider what is attainable for your body type or somatotype.

What's Your Body Type?

The term *somatotype* was coined by W.H. Sheldon in the 1940s as a way to characterize the three principal human forms: endomorphic (endomorphs), mesomorphic (mesomorphs), and ectomorphic (ectomorphs). Sheldon named the three primary body types after three germ layers associated with embryonic development. Some of his original theories were not sound (i.e., theories related to psychological temperament based on your physique), and scientists later disproved them, but his classifications have merit from a human biological perspective.

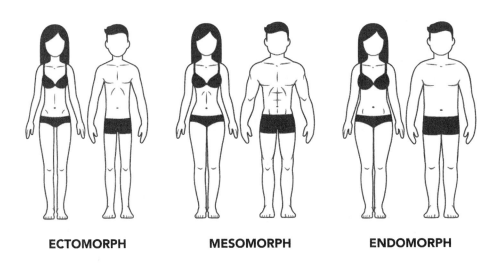

ECTOMORPH   **MESOMORPH**   **ENDOMORPH**

Each somatotype reacts to weight gain and loss in different ways. Nutritionists, trainers, doctors, and other health professionals utilize somatotypes to create customized training and nutrition protocols. All body types can gain or lose weight, but the degree and rate at which they do so vary.

- ECTOMORPHS tend to be long and lean and may struggle to gain weight or muscle.
- MESOMORPHS are naturally muscular and tend to easily gain or lose weight.
- ENDOMORPHS tend to be pear-shaped, easily store fat, and may have a difficult time losing weight.

Not everyone fits into a single category; some have qualities of two body types or more. However, while we may not fit an exact body type, we will fit into one category better than the others.

So why create a plan based on body types? One answer: realistic expectations. Clients often bring me a photo of someone they saw online and ask me to make their body look a certain way. Body types provide context to show people what types of changes are achievable through proper training and nutrition.

Discovering the various body types and learning my own was a pivotal moment in my life. I felt seen. I felt understood. Body typing made sense because it described my reality. I easily gained and lost weight. I knew I was a mesomorph; it described me to a T. I had friends who were ectomorphs and could eat much more than I could, yet never struggled with their weight.

This understanding was crucial to my success with clients, too. When I worked with clients who gained weight easily and struggled to lose it (aka endomorphs), I witnessed their struggle firsthand. I worked with them, side by side, day by day, week by week, and witnessed 100-percent compliance to a plan that just did not produce the same results. Coaching opened my eyes to the necessity of customization: What worked for me didn't work for everyone.

Eating for Your Macro Type

The body-typing approach is an excellent starting point but falls short because someone's physical appearance doesn't always dictate how they should be eating. As a nutritionist, there is no way I can write a nutrition plan that will apply to each client based merely on body type, because there are too many nuances to consider outside of body type alone. The biggest variable is carb tolerance level, which I will cover in great detail in Chapter 4.

General body-typing guidelines advise endomorphs to eat fewer carbs, tell mesomorphs to be moderate in carbs, and say that ectomorphs do best with high-carb approaches. This is way too general, as there are hormonal and metabolic factors that have significant impacts on one's appropriate macronutrient ratios. Anecdotal evidence from body typing alone is an unreliable gauge to guide anyone with respect to nutrition.

This is where I came up with the concept of eating for your macro type, a profile based on your body type and other factors, such as your tolerance to carbs. While body typing is a suitable gauge to tailor training protocols, it isn't the best guide on how to eat, because it doesn't consider your biochemical response to the three different macronutrients, especially carbohydrates.

UNLOCKING YOUR MACRO TYPE:
REAL STORIES, REAL SUCCESSES

Marianna, Carb-Fueled Macro Type

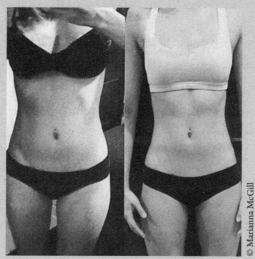

© Marianna McGill

Before   *After*

Get inspired by one of my all-time favorite carb-dominant transformations: Marianna was eating only about 1,100 calories per day. She is a medical device sales person, so she is on her feet and in and out of hospitals all day. An ectomorph with a naturally lean physique, Marianna struggles to gain weight but wanted to lean out her torso and show more definition in her stomach. People tell her all the time that she already looks great and doesn't need to lose weight. But for her, she wanted a more defined physique. She was shocked when I upped her calories to 2,500 a day, favoring carbohydrates. She was even more shocked to see her waist get smaller and smaller week after week in spite of the increased carbs. This is a classic example of how not eating enough carbs can actually interfere with your ability to drop body fat. She gained weight during this program, but she gained lean muscle and dropped body fat. In six weeks she lost 3.5 inches off her waistline. She gained tremendous strength during the program and had substantially more energy than ever before.

There is much debate in the nutrition community over the best way to fuel the body — from lower-fat, carb-fueled plans to diets that are extremely low in carbs and high in fat. The first plan that really worked for me was a protein-fueled macronutrient approach, common to fitness competitors and bodybuilders. I ate a diet that was high in protein, low in fat, and moderate in carbs. This led to my own breakthrough in my fat-loss journey and helped me discover the key that allowed my clients to experience similar results.

Over the last decade, I've learned that while this plan worked for me, it won't work for everyone; it will work for some, just not *all*. This is why I have dedicated my career to identifying solutions for those who are trying what's popular and feeling defeated.

If you feel stuck, I feel your pain because I, too, was stuck, frustrated, and extremely confused for almost half of my life. I tried all of the popular diet plans only to realize that if a diet is popular, that means it worked for the author of that book and its followers, not that it's right for you. This book will provide you with the macronutrient formula that's tailor-made for you, and will not force you into yet another one-size-fits-most program that doesn't work for *you*.

While you may never aspire to look like a bodybuilder, there are key takeaways from a traditional bodybuilder's diet that, when applied properly, can lead to incredible physique changes. Many are blown away by how much *more* protein they need to consume compared to the USDA's standards of 10 percent of your total calories, or 50 grams per day on a 2,000-calorie-per-day diet. That recommendation is based on the amount of nitrogen the body needs for DNA resynthesis and doesn't account for the amount needed to support lean muscle mass development and targeted fat loss.

My recommendations for protein intake are much higher than the USDA's 50 grams per day (or 10 percent of your total caloric intake or 0.36 g/kg). For protein-dominant macro types, my recommendations can be anywhere from 120 grams or more per day for women and 170 grams or more per day for men (or 1 to 1.2 grams per pound of lean muscle mass). When in a caloric deficit, high-protein intake paired with intense training supports an increase in lean muscle tissue and boosts fat loss of stored body fat.[1] Protein is the only macronutrient that contains nitrogen. When your body is in a positive nitrogen balance, it allows you to use fat for fuel while sparing lean muscle tissue. This enables you to drop fat while boosting lean muscle definition for a fit and athletic physique. High-protein nutrition protocols tend to be low in fat and moderate in carbohydrates.

As noted earlier, there's much debate in the nutrition community about the best way to fuel your body. Some individuals thrive using plans that are high in carbs, others need more fats, and others need more protein. This doesn't mean that high-fat diets are bad just because a low-fat diet is what works for you; it doesn't mean that a low-carb diet is bad because moderate carbs work in your case; and it doesn't mean that everyone needs more protein. When my first endomorph client didn't respond to the protein-fueled approach that was working so well for me, I manipulated her macros by dialing down the carbs while increasing her dietary fats. Once I made this shift, we started to see not only her body change but also her energy levels. This challenged everything I'd experienced with regard to fat loss. It meant that some people performed better when more of their calories came from fat as opposed to carbs. But why? The answer, I would come to find out, is carb tolerance.

The Missing Key: Carb Tolerance

Carb tolerance is exactly what it sounds like: a measurement of how many carbs are appropriate for your body and your diet. Understanding your personal carb tolerance can be a game-changer when it comes to your health, wellness, and fitness goals.

The reality is, there are varying degrees of carb tolerance. This became evident to me when I observed more and more clients — of varying body types — who were not able to reduce body fat or drop weight or inches when a high portion of their total calories came from carbohydrates, even when in a caloric deficit. The more clients I worked with, the more I realized that they weren't outliers and that carb tolerance needed to be a solid consideration before assigning one's macros.

Here's the problem: The USDA recommends 60 to 65 percent of our total calories come from carbohydrates on a diet of 2,000 calories per day. This translates into roughly 300 grams of carbs a day. The type of person who can effectively follow this nutrition approach is a Carb-Fueled Macro Type, meaning they can get a significant amount of their calories from carbohydrates and still lose fat. This is a terrible starting point for the average person looking to improve their body composition, because only a fraction of the population can actually eat this way and thrive.

Some think that they only gain fat when they eat too much food. Not true. **The biggest factor that dictates how you should eat for your macro type is how your body responds to carbohydrates.** If you have ever wondered why some people seem to gain weight just by looking at carbs while others can eat all the carbs they want and never gain a pound, it is because people process carbohydrates differently. I know it's not fair, but some metabolic types have a higher carb tolerance than others. Once you grasp the science behind your carb tolerance level, you can navigate your health journey with a clear understanding of the most appropriate way to fuel your body.

UNLOCKING YOUR MACRO TYPE:
REAL STORIES, REAL SUCCESSES

Michelle, Fat-Fueled Macro Type

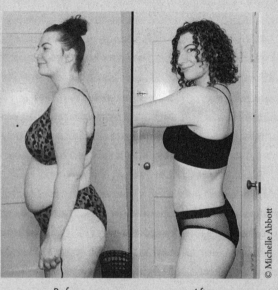

Before   *After*

Michelle is an insulin-resistant mesomorph. Most other plans would have her eating higher carbs than she can actually tolerate. She's a mesomorph with a relatively even distribution of body fat, yet she can't tolerate carbs the way other mesomorphs can. To achieve her 40-pound weight loss, she switched between keto and low-carb/high-fat plans and ultimately ended up experiencing a more sustainable lifestyle on the low-carb/high-fat eating style. She was able to drop inches everywhere with more ease than on conventional higher-carb plans, has felt better than ever, doesn't feel restricted, and actually looks forward to her meals!

Your carb tolerance is based on your body's sensitivity to insulin. Insulin is a hormone that shuttles glucose and amino acids into your cells to give them energy while supporting muscle growth. You have a tipping point for carb intake where carb consumption is *good* and helps you build muscle and gives you energy to perform at your highest level. The problem is, when carb intake exceeds your body's energy requirements plus your carb storage limits, insulin becomes a fat-storing hormone. This is why some individuals can eat carbs while maintaining lean muscle mass and low levels of body fat and some can't. The body can store carbs in the muscle cells, in the liver, and in the blood. The average healthy adult can store around 500 to 550 grams of carbs with 80 to 90 percent of them being in the muscle cells, 5 to 10 percent in the liver, and a small amount in the bloodstream. When you consume more than this threshold *and* are inactive, your body hits a tipping point where insulin will take the excess carbs it can't use and convert them to fat to use as energy later on.

The body can hold on to only so many carbs. If those carbs aren't going to be used in the cells for energy, they are going to be stored as fat. The body has an unlimited ability to store body fat but a finite ability to store carbs.

All carbs are not created equal. It's easy to overshoot your carb intake if you are used to consuming processed foods with empty sugars. For instance, a sweet Starbucks coffee beverage can contain well over 60 grams of carbs, with 100 percent of those carbs coming from sugar, leaving you with no sense of fullness or satisfaction. However, if you were to consume 60 grams of carbs from high-fiber vegetables like zucchini, you'd have to eat a total of 15 cups at 4 grams of carbs per cup. It probably wouldn't take 15 cups of vegetables for you to feel full. This is why it's crucial to be mindful of not only how many carbs you consume in a day but also the *type* of carbs. Many people blow their daily carb budget on foods that do not fill them up.

How many carbs one can consume varies from person to person based on your overall carb tolerance, how much exercise you get, and how much energy your activity levels demand. Think of athletes like Michael Phelps or LeBron James, who burn thousands of calories a day in practice to maintain their current mass. Most people underestimate how many carbs they consume while overestimating how many calories they burn. This is a recipe for disaster, and I see clients make this mistake over and over again. You're better off being more conservative by underestimating your calories burned and overestimating food intake. If you consume more carbs than you burn and you aren't performing resistance training to a level that challenges your muscles to grow, insulin will convert these excess carbs to stored body fat for future energy use. Higher carb intake without the addition of proper resistance training exercises will not result in muscle gain.

Macros: A Science-Backed Approach

Over the last ten years, working with tens of thousands of clients, I've classified the most common nutrition-based solutions into five primary categories, an approach I call *macro typing*. Macro typing is a simple way to characterize the nature of the most suitable nutrition strategy for an individual.

Your macro type is a bio-individual nutrition blueprint that enables you to function and feel your best. This book will reveal your macro type, or the predominant macronutrient — protein, carbohydrate, or fat — your body needs. This sets the foundation for how to balance your nutritional needs to support your health goals. If you've been frustrated by diet plan after diet plan, it's most likely because those programs weren't aligned with your macro type. Maybe they were too low-carb for you or too high in fat. Maybe they lacked sufficient protein. The beauty of using macros is that you consider the chemical composition of the foods you consume, allowing you to make an informed choice based on science, not speculation.

As a scientist, when I look at a food, I consider what it is made of, how that will break down in the body, and how I am going to measure its properties. The chemical engineer in me is always looking for ways to quantify the physical, chemical, nutritional, and organoleptic properties of foods. I do this because I have a background in quality control in research and development and food manufacturing. You may see a food, but I see a pH range, a moisture content range, a percentage of protein, an ash content, a mesh size (the overall particle size of certain powders), amounts of certain kinds of fat (saturated fat, trans fat, etc.) . . . and the list goes on.

For example, where you see an egg, I see 5 grams of fat and 6.5 grams of protein. You see a banana; I see 25 grams of carbs. I don't see the food; I see the composition. Think of it like learning a new language: It may feel foreign at first, but the more you practice it, the better you get. Once you become aware of the macro compositions of foods, you have precise information to see exactly what is stopping you from reaching your goals.

Whether you keep track or not, you eat a certain number of calories per day, and those calories are made up of either proteins, carbs, or fats. Eating without understanding macros is like shopping without checking price tags. Imagine going to the store and purchasing whatever merchandise you want without knowing what it costs. By the time your credit card statement comes around, you'd be in complete shock. No matter your budget, knowing the price is essential to consider before adding something to your cart.

So why on earth would you not do the same when it comes to foods? You're not going to be successful if you eat with zero consideration of the protein, carb, and fat content of your meals.

When it comes down to it, weight loss — scientifically backed weight loss — isn't that complicated. In order to lose weight, you need to consume fewer calories than you need to sustain your current body mass. However, eating at a caloric deficit won't improve your body composition unless you are intentional about the quality of those calories. Sure, eating "less" will keep you from gaining weight, but it won't necessarily drop your body fat, increase your lean muscle mass, or create a significant change in your overall shape.

If you are like I once was, you may be overly obsessed with the number on the scale. Just because you are losing weight doesn't mean you're experiencing "quality" weight loss. **Weight loss and fat loss are not the same thing.** If you get upset when the scale doesn't go down, or if it only goes down a little, you may be missing the improvements in your body composition that don't always translate into weight loss. When you see the number on the scale go down, it could be a combination of water, muscle, or fat loss. Ideally, you want to hold on to your muscle and drop only stored body fat. You can still be holding on to excess body fat even if you are at a low body weight. This results in a body composition that, while smaller overall, may still not be lean in appearance (this is often referred to as *skinny fat*). In order to target fat loss, the *composition* of the calories you consume actually matters. Weight loss isn't always a "good" thing, and weight gain isn't a "bad" thing at all if you are dropping body fat and gaining lean muscle.

Trust in the Plan, and Give It Time to Work

Ever since I started making YouTube videos, I've been blown away by how many people don't know how to properly approach their nutrition. At the same time, I'm not surprised, because I was once one of them — completely frustrated with the process, disappointed in my physique, and desperate for results. When you reach this level of desperation, you're tempted to throw all logic out the window, because you literally just want to get any sign that you are actually seeing a change in your body, no matter how extreme or how crazy the new plan is. This process can take a huge mental and emotional toll, leaving you feeling tired, hungry, socially isolated, on edge, and lacking quality of life. I know, I've been there. And it saddens me to see people still suffering and frustrated like this, because there's a much better way.

The biggest problem I've observed over the last decade is that people tend to correlate an arbitrary reduction of calories to be equivalent to eating properly. It's typically either all or nothing: the eat "all the things" and screw the gym mindset, or the eat-next-to-nothing while working out like a maniac mindset. *Neither* is a practical solution.

There is a healthy way to do this, a way that won't starve you, that yields measurable results, and that allows you to feel better in your skin while working toward your goals. I encourage my clients to stop fighting the process, because there really are no shortcuts if you want lasting and meaningful results.

You didn't gain that excess body fat overnight. It accumulated over the course of days, weeks, months, and in some cases years. Every time you ate excess calories, those extra calories were like purchases made on a credit card. You didn't need to pay for it right then and there, but if you didn't pay off your credit card once a month, you owed what you spent, plus interest — and that can add up quickly.

Overeating is similar. Each time you overeat, your body doesn't just forget it. Those extra calories will stay with you until you burn them off. It's all fun and games, eating and drinking whatever you feel like, until it's time to face the music and pay the bill. If you're reading this, you may have been racking up this food debt for *years.* Just as you wouldn't expect to pay off credit card debt that you have been accumulating for years in just a few weeks, you shouldn't expect to burn tens of thousands of calories (or even hundreds of thousands of calories) in just a few weeks.

Once you're past denial and are ready to face your reality, you must accept two truths:

1. This is not going to happen overnight.
2. This journey may not look like what you expected.

UNLOCKING YOUR MACRO TYPE: REAL STORIES, REAL SUCCESSES

Delilah, Protein-Fueled Macro Type

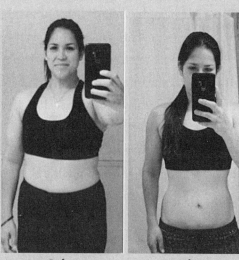

Before   *After*

© Delilah Gonzalez

Delilah came to me ready to commit to her health. She was already strong and athletic and took martial arts and boxing classes regularly, but her nutrition was lacking. She is a mesomorph body type who gains weight relatively evenly on her frame and loses it with ease when dialed in. She is a Protein-Fueled Macro Type with moderate carb tolerance. This means that she didn't need to go insanely low carb to make progress; she was able to maintain a moderate carb intake of between 100 and 150 grams while going high in protein and low in fat. The biggest adjustment she experienced was learning how to hit her protein macros. This meant adapting to foods that are higher in protein and lower in fat. She swapped whole eggs for egg whites, transitioned to leaner meats, more veggies, and lower-sugar fruit, and added protein supplements as needed. She never felt hungry, dropped from 34 to 27 inches in her waist, and has been able to keep it off for a year!

Some of you might be shocked to learn that you need to eat much more of specific nutrients like protein or fat, which may feel like a lot more food than you thought you needed. For others, you may find that you are overdoing it on certain nutrients, and as a result your progress has stalled. Embrace this opportunity to learn, and don't cringe at the harsh truths that you will uncover during this process. Instead, acknowledge the power in becoming educated about your body, about nutrition, and about the pieces you've been missing all along.

So where do we begin? To start, we need to identify three things:

1. The number of calories you need to be consuming for your goal
2. Your carb tolerance level
3. Your predominant macro type

Your calories tell us how much of a deficit you need to lose weight. Your carb tolerance level will illuminate whether you'll have the most success on a low-, medium-, or higher-carb diet. And your macro type will help us gauge the most appropriate macronutrient breakdown of those calories and the best exercise and training methods for your body.

Most people have no idea what a proper day of eating should look like. Most are in denial about how much they are eating. Even those who make sincere efforts to be mindful of eating healthfully may not realize how many calories they are taking in, what nutrients they are missing, and how the breakdown of their food intake impacts their physique. Even if you only shop at farmers' markets, buy all organic food, and make a conscious effort to consume healthy ingredients, it's not necessarily going to lead to fat loss. And that's frustrating! Not only are you worried about eating too much, but you're also wondering: *Is this okay? Is that okay? What am I looking for? How do I know?*

UNLOCKING YOUR MACRO TYPE: REAL STORIES, REAL SUCCESSES

Pam, Protein-Fueled/Low-Carb Macro Type

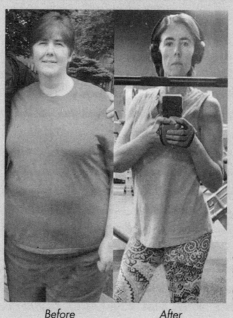

© Pam Snyder

Before   *After*

I've had the pleasure of working with Pam for over a year and a half. After taking my mastering macros certification course, she went on to become a member of my team and now helps me help others. She overcame thyroid cancer and a stroke. She was given months to live and chose to fight for her life. It wasn't until she found the macros approach that she was able to take her progress to the next level. Before finding this program, she tried it all: from veganism (high-carb, low-fat) to Atkins, and everything in between. She didn't feel good on any other plan. She needed practical tools to gauge and measure not only her progress with fat loss but also how the plan made her feel. Other plans left her feeling completely and utterly drained. What mattered the most to Pam was improving the quality of her life. She's lost 130 pounds by eating real whole foods and staying mindful of the *why* behind her journey. She inspires everyone she touches, and it's been an honor and privilege to witness her transformation.

The good news is there is a simpler way to navigate this dilemma.

Instead of viewing nutrition with regard to what you need to eliminate, you will experience far more success focusing on both the macro- and micronutrients that you need. No diet is inherently bad; you just need to match it to *your* macro type.

But first, I want to explain more to you about fat so you can understand what it is, where it goes, and why it can be so hard to lose.

2

The Secret Code of Fat

Body fat is one of the most misunderstood topics in the health and fitness space. Most resources only provide superficial information that fails to connect some very important dots. Once you understand these dots, you can master your own fat loss like never before.

You probably already know that body fat is a source of stored energy. But you might not be aware that it's also an endocrine organ, and that your body stores it in various forms for different purposes. Understanding where the body stores body fat and why is foundational to transforming it. Once you learn *why* it won't budge, you can get to the business of reversing the trend.

Since you are reading this book, you are seeking practical, science-based answers as to why you are experiencing the challenges you are. Addressing the circumstances that are causing your body fat to hang around does not need to feel like you are trying to solve a Rubik's Cube. To crack the fat code, you only need to understand what fat actually is, the different types, and which factors impact where it is stored.

Most people think of fat as something bad that they need to get rid of. That thinking is flawed. Before you wish all your fat away, recognize that fat is an essential element of human function. The real goal should be learning to sustain a healthy amount of body fat. Fat is *not* the enemy. In fact, adipose tissue (aka fat) is a metabolically active organ. You don't think of your heart or intestines as organs that you need to get rid of, so don't ever think you need to eliminate fat entirely. Your adipose tissue doesn't just make your pants too tight; it plays an important role in your body.

In the last few decades, research has revealed that fat cells play an essential role in recognizing and responding to fluctuations in systemic energy balance.[1] Fat, the largest endocrine organ in the human body, releases a multitude of chemical messengers and has an unlimited ability to expand throughout the course of your life.[2]

The body's built-in biological adaptation mechanism to store fat was once a key to surviving long periods when food was scarce. Now, it is the bane of about two-thirds of Americans who are overweight or obese.[3] Fat loss presents a challenge in a world where calorie-dense, nutrient-poor foods are more abundant than ever. And since the body is hormonally programmed to store fat in times of abundance (just in case food later becomes scarce), we all have a natural biological tendency to store fat.

Four Main Types of Body Fat

There are four primary types of fat in the body, and they each play a different — and important — role in health and demand special consideration when it comes to fat loss.

ESSENTIAL FAT

Essential fat is the minimum threshold to support basic physiological functions, below which human life is not sustainable. You *need* a certain amount of body fat to support reproduction and other vital functions. Essential fat is located in places from bone marrow to lipid-rich tissues that support the central nervous system to vital organs like the heart, kidneys, lungs, liver, spleen, and intestines. As stated by the American

Council on Exercise, women require a body composition of at least 10 to 13 percent essential fat and men require a minimum of 2 to 5 percent to support vital functions such as vitamin absorption, temperature regulation, and fertility.[4]

In order to see visible six-pack abs, a female needs to be less than about 13 percent body fat, where a male needs to be under 10 percent. It's common to see female fitness competitors drop below their essential levels of body fat, which results in missed periods (known as *amenorrhea*). And in the months leading up to competitions, female fitness competitors can even drop under 10 percent body fat, whereas male bodybuilders may drop to as low as 3 percent. Being shredded 24/7, 365 is not recommended, nor is it sustainable.

Having visible abs does not mean you are "healthy," although social media will lead you to believe otherwise. Even with a remarkable figure, fitness competitors and bodybuilders do not necessarily possess the best possible body composition. Going all out to attain this level of leanness may compromise your athletic performance, increase fatigue, heighten your risk of injury, impair your body's ability to regulate temperature, and put your body in a catabolic state where you will lose calorie-burning muscle tissue. Reducing body fat is a great way to increase your sports performance, but don't overdo it by taking your body below its essential body fat requirements.

Common signs of hormone imbalances related to low body fat levels include overdependence on caffeine, extreme fatigue, hair loss, poor sleep quality, feeling cold, brain fog, difficulty concentrating, anxiety, digestion issues, prolonged muscle soreness, and reduced recovery rate, to name a few.

Never lose your health in the mission to be healthy. It is estimated that over 45 percent of athletic females deal with menstrual irregularity or missed cycles. Just because this is happening does not mean it is *normal!* This issue is due to a combination of your body fat levels approaching the minimum level of essential body fat coupled with a reduced availability of energy (due to overtraining, undereating, or both). Females experiencing the loss of their monthly cycle as a result of body fat being at or below the essential level, overtraining, or a caloric deficit exceeding 800 calories per day will begin to experience low levels of the leptin hormone, a sign of hormonal imbalance (see Leptin: The Satiety Hormone, below).

If one remains at or below the essential level of body fat required for functional health, it can reduce the body's ability to absorb the fat-soluble vitamins A, D, E, and K. Going too low in essential body fat may lead to nutrient deficiencies, electrolyte imbalances, gastrointestinal issues, immune system irregularities, internal organ shrinkage, nervous system damage, starvation, and even death. The bottom line? Do not mess with your essential body fat levels.

LEPTIN: THE SATIETY HORMONE

Leptin is a hormone produced by fat cells that tells your brain to stop eating when you're full.[5] It would seem logical that if you have excess fat, you'd make more leptin, be less hungry, and as a result get back to your optimal weight, but that's not the case.

When you have excess leptin, your cells become leptin-resistant! This means that it's even harder for your brain to get the message that you're full, so you end up eating more! This is a situation where "willpower" won't work because your body is resisting the message that you are full on a cellular level.

When your body fat is below essential requirements, your reproductive hormonal health is compromised. Humans respond to famine by directing energy toward surviving and away from reproducing. Scientists found that reduced leptin levels due to starvation played a crucial role in regulating hormonal responses.[6] About 70 percent of women between the ages of 18 and 35 who stopped getting their period due to hormonal abnormalities were able to start ovulation again after receiving daily leptin injections.[7] This shows that leptin levels can serve as indicators of imbalances and when adjusted to their proper level can enable one to regulate and re-establish a regular monthly cycle.

Scientists have proven that leptin levels respond in proportion to changes in certain macronutrients. Their studies demonstrated that carbohydrates create a more significant increase in leptin levels than fat. This means raising carbohydrate intake can support an increase in leptin levels, which is necessary in order to restore a regular monthly cycle. It also means periodically raising one's carbohydrate intake is an effective means of preventing leptin levels from going too low. This is crucial to supporting hormonal health, especially in women.

SUBCUTANEOUS FAT

If you have ever ordered a steak at a restaurant and seen a layer of fat around the perimeter of the meat, that is subcutaneous fat. Subcutaneous fat describes fat on top of muscle tissue under the surface of the skin. Any fat you can see or pinch on your body is subcutaneous. It serves as a protective layer of insulation as well as a cushion from intense trauma. It's also what most of us focus on when we're trying to shed fat. While you may want to get rid of subcutaneous fat for aesthetic purposes, this type of fat does not necessarily put your health at risk. It's not as dangerous as the intra-abdominal fat that surrounds your organs known as visceral fat (see page 30). Subcutaneous fat layers will be the first you burn as fuel on a fat-loss program, before your body goes after visceral fat.

When I work with clients in person, I calculate subcutaneous fat with the caliper method, which measures targeted skin folds in the abdominal, thigh, back, and upper arm regions. We then plug these values into a mathematical model to estimate body fat percentage, lean mass, and fat mass. According to the American Council on Exercise, ideal body fat percentage ranges for women and men are as follows:

TARGET BODY FAT PERCENTAGE RANGES FOR WOMEN & MEN

Category	Female Body Fat %	Male Body Fat %
Ultra-lean	10–13	2–5
Athletic	14–20	6–13
Fit	21–24	14–17
Healthy	25–31	18–24
Obese	>32	>25

The purpose of this chart is to provide practical parameters around body fat percentage ranges to get an idea of your current body fat level relative to your target range. This information is crucial to get a feel for how long it will take you to reach your goal based on the assumption that one can lose approximately 0.5 percent body fat per week. When selecting your target body fat percentage, keep in mind that ultra-lean is in the range for essential fat, so it is the bare minimum people need to sustain vital functionality. You can see from this chart that the essential fat level required by females is significantly higher than it is for men, but it is also in the range of most professional female fitness competitors. It is advised to NOT go below the essential body fat ranges. Athletes will be at a slightly higher body fat range with 14 to 20 percent for women and 6 to 13 percent for men. The majority of fit individuals who work out regularly and sustain a healthy diet will be in the range of 21 to 24 percent for women and 14 to 17 percent for men. For general health, it is advised to be between 25 and 31 percent for women and 18 and 24 percent for men. Anything higher than 32 percent for women and 25 percent for men is considered obese.

When it comes to subcutaneous fat, it tends to feel soft and have a fluffy appearance, so when you lose it, you can also drop a dress size (or several). That said, less fat doesn't always correlate with a lower number on the scale. For example, if you train for strength, you can gain muscle while you lose fat, so your body weight might be the same even though you now wear a smaller size.

You cannot spot-reduce subcutaneous fat. Expect to lose it from the parts of your body with the highest concentrations of fat first. Your hormones and genetics are responsible for dictating your personal fat distribution pattern. For women, this tends to be the chest, waist, hips, and thighs. For men, it's the waist. Based on my experience as a health coach since 2010, if you are less than 250 pounds and following this program by eating in a caloric deficit according to your macros and working out a minimum of four times a week, you can expect to lose up to ½ inch (1.27 cm) off the smallest part of your waist per week. If you weigh more than 250 pounds, you may lose up to 1 inch (2.54 cm) off your waist per week, maybe slightly more in the first seven to ten days.

INTRAMUSCULAR FAT

Fatty muscles? Is this an actual thing? Yes. Intramuscular fat (IMF) is an ectopic deposit of fat embedded within the muscle fibers. This type of fat forms as skeletal muscle fibers sandwich liquid droplets of fat next to your mitochondria, for the cells to use as a source of energy for physical activity. This makes it very easy for your body to access and utilize during exercise, because your muscles can utilize fatty acids as fuel. This means that during a workout, your body taps IMF for energy first. It's harder to access and more challenging to metabolize the majority of your fat, because the body stores it in stubborn regions with little to no blood flow. For instance, of all the fat on your thigh, only 8 percent is IMF. The rest is subcutaneous.[8]

There is a strong link between carb tolerance levels and overall mobility. This is due to the accumulation of inflamed cells concentrated around intramuscular fat deposits. When muscles are inflamed, it is harder for the muscle cells to metabolize carbohydrates. If your muscles can't process the carbs you are eating due to excess inflammation from localized fat within the muscle, it can actually lead to the onset of insulin resistance.[9] IMF alone can lead to a serious reduction in muscle metabolism, resulting in reduced carb tolerance levels compared to an individual with little to no intramuscular fat deposits. IMF serves as a meaningful gauge of mobility and muscle function as we age, in both range of motion and ability to get around. Too much IMF introduces inflammation, making it more physically challenging to move about freely.

So, what causes higher levels of IMF? Inactivity is one of the major causes. Immobilizing injuries can increase IMF content as much as 25 percent in only three months' time. This means that prolonged periods of inactivity can easily reverse all your hard work to gain muscle and lose fat. If that's not motivation to get moving, I don't know what is!

Higher levels of this type of fat are related to reduced strength in older women.[10] In another study, researchers found that age is a strong factor in determining the likelihood of IMF in both women and men, regardless of whether one gained, lost, or experienced no change in weight.[11] This goes to show, weight loss alone won't improve your body fat as you age. However, resistance training can lower IMF in individuals over 55.[12] This is an important consideration for those who choose to remain scale-obsessed. It's a rude awakening, seeing that even at a lower body weight, your IMF does not decline. Our society has placed far too much emphasis on body weight as a marker of health. In reality, body composition (i.e., muscle mass, body fat, bone density, etc.) is a better indicator.

One way to better understand IMF and what causes it is to look at the agricultural industry. While we want lower IMF, the cattle industry spends millions in research and development learning how to increase bovine IMF. This produces highly marbled, more valuable meat (think rib eye). These fat deposits within the muscle are the direct result of the bovine diet. Cattle ranchers and farmers feed their livestock a high-calorie, high-carb diet, the majority of which is corn, with the intention of producing marbling (aka IMF) in the meat. Livestock in the U.S. yields meat with 6 to 8 percent fat after being on this nutrition regimen for a year or so. In Japan, cattle ranches and farms are able to yield beef (aka Wagyu) with IMF in the range of 30 to 35 percent, with the main difference being the fact that their cows are on a high-calorie, high-carb diet for a longer period of time (three years or more). It's important to note, the entire meat industry utilizes a high-calorie, high-carb diet for animals based on its ability to produce higher-fat meat. When we eat in a similar fashion, we end up with high levels of IMF, insulin resistance, and type 2 diabetes.

The good news is that IMF is responsive to exercise, weight training in particular. Most active individuals tend to be insulin-sensitive, meaning they can process insulin without issue, and the body is responsive to messenger signals regarding how it is metabolizing glucose. Boosting your activity and making a simple macronutrient ratio shift away from a very high-carb diet is essential to lowering IMF.

The presence of IMF isn't necessarily a bad thing, but small amounts can be early warning signs of more troublesome issues down the road.

VISCERAL FAT

This kind of fat is unique because the body stores it deep within the abdominal cavity, beneath the abdominal muscles, in close proximity to vital organs such as the stomach, intestines, liver, and heart. Visceral fat is composed of biologically active cells that secrete both hormones and inflammatory molecules.[13] These hormones disrupt your body's natural patterns for processing both dietary fats and carbohydrates. The number one sign of visceral fat is concentrated fat in the torso, which is crudely measured by waist circumference. Abdominal obesity is the concentrated accumulation of visceral fat in the torso.

About 10 percent of all body fat is visceral fat. (The remaining 90 percent is subcutaneous.) The most accurate ways to measure visceral fat are using an MRI or CT scan, but those tests are costly. The next best way to gauge if you are at risk for more than 10 percent of your total fat coming from visceral fat is to measure the circumference of the largest portion of your waist. If your waist is greater than 35 inches (88.9 cm) for a woman or 40 inches (101.6 cm) for a man, you are at an increased risk.

In addition to measuring your torso, another useful calculation is the waist-to-hip ratio (WHR). To get this ratio, measure the smallest part of your waist and divide it by the largest part of your hips. The World Health Organization (WHO) utilizes the WHR as a gauge of visceral adiposity. For a frame of reference, the anatomical WHR for a natural female hourglass figure with a waistline smaller than the hips (think Halle Berry) is 0.7. The closer this value is to 1, the more the midsection protrudes, and the greater the health risk.

HEALTH RISK LEVEL RELATED TO WAIST
TO HIP RATIOS IN WOMEN & MEN

HEALTH RISK	WOMEN	MEN
Low	<0.80	<0.90
Moderate	0.80–0.85	0.90–0.95
High	>0.85	>0.95

This chart indexes the level of associated health risk in women and men based on the waist to hip ratio, which is the circumference of the smallest part of the waist in inches divided by the largest part of the hips in inches. This allows for clearer interpretation of your relative health risk based on how much visceral fat you are carrying on your frame. Health risk level is based on the correlation of visceral fat content with high cholesterol, type 2 diabetes, stroke, and heart disease. Visceral fat contributes to the narrowing of your blood vessels and causes inflammation of internal organs and tissues. A pear-shape female body type tends to have more subcutaneous fat compared to an apple-shape type, which is likely to have more visceral fat.

High concentrations of fat in the torso as a result of accumulated visceral fat tends to be more common in men. If you have ever seen a rounded potbelly with a hard texture (compared to the soft texture of subcutaneous fat), you have seen visceral fat. This fat is rock hard due to its proximity to the organs. The fat itself is not hard per se; it's tightly packed as deposits between the organs, resulting in a rigid feeling since this type of fat is concentrated beneath the walls of the abdomen. This results in a very dense rounded core.

Because we have different types of fat that live in different parts of our body, it is important to understand the different risks they carry. Whether you have 5 pounds to lose or more than 100, it's crucial to be aware of the high-risk zone for visceral fat concentration and the state of your current health in relation to that danger zone.

UNLOCKING YOUR MACRO TYPE: REAL STORIES, REAL SUCCESSES

Jessica, Fat-Fueled/Low-Carb Macro Type

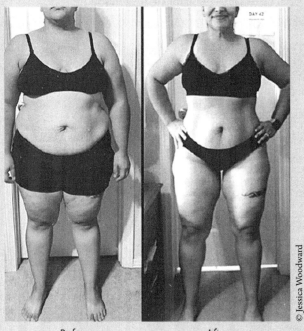

Before   After

Jessica has a classic endomorph body and gains weight easily but struggles to lose weight. The mother of three boys, she has her hands full from the moment she opens her eyes to the moment she closes them. She came to me weighing over 235 pounds. We learned very quickly that her body thrives on higher fats and lower carbs; not only does she lose weight with more ease on this approach, but it helps stabilize her energy, keeps her focused, keeps her mentally alert, and curbs her cravings. She is completely satisfied on this eating style and was surprised to learn that she could enjoy her food this much and still lose weight! She has lost over 50 pounds and believes that eating for her macro type is the only way that works for her needs and busy lifestyle.

Age, genetics, nutrition, activity, and hormones all impact body fat. You cannot change age or genetics. You *can* do something about nutrition and activity, which you will learn more about later in this book. However, at the end of the day, hormones drive fat storage, and age and genetics are major factors in how they do so. If you have been perplexed your whole life as to why fat accumulates in specific areas, understanding how hormones drive this behavior is the answer.

Hormones and Body Fat

Hormones, specifically sex hormones, play a big role in the way the body stores fat at various stages of your life. Your body fat distribution is related to hormonal changes dating all the way back to puberty.

ESTROGEN

Estrogen is the primary sex hormone that drives a woman's body to change over the course of her life. Men have estrogen as well but at much lower levels. Most of this hormone's production takes place in the ovaries (testes in men), adrenals, and fat cells (yes, your fat cells create estrogen). There are three types of estrogen: estradiol, estrone, and estriol. For the purpose of this book, we are most concerned with the influence of estradiol, as estrone is associated with menopause and estriol is associated with pregnancy. Estradiol drives changes in the reproductive system.

Before puberty, males and females have about the same amount of estradiol. For women, puberty begins when the brain signals the ovaries to start producing estrogen, which raises estradiol levels.

The spike in these hormones happens around puberty, when a woman first gets her period and reaches sexual maturity.[14] This results in an average weight gain of about 15 pounds over a period of two to four years, with an average body fat level of about 20 to 25 percent in healthy adolescent females. During puberty, increased levels of estrogen result in the buildup of subcutaneous fat. Keep in mind, these are still healthy levels of body fat.

The problem arises when subcutaneous body fat increases as a result of weight gain, causing estrogen levels to rise. Fat tissue also creates and stores estrogen. This results in a hormone imbalance known as *estrogen dominance*. It then becomes a chicken-or-egg scenario regarding which came first: Is there more estrogen because of higher fat levels or more fat because of high estrogen? The reality is, it's a combination of both.

Estrogen Dominance

While the term *estrogen dominance* may seem like it describes a women's empowerment movement, this is something no woman wants to experience.

Symptoms of estrogen dominance include mood swings, weight gain (in the chest, waist, and hips), very light or extremely heavy periods, fibrocystic breasts, uterine fibroids, anxiety, sugar cravings, low libido, irritability, depression, joint pain, and body aches. Health risks associated with estrogen dominance include hormonal cancers (breast, uterine, ovarian, and prostate), autoimmune diseases, candida overgrowth, and thyroid dysfunction. To top it off, estrogen dominance makes exercise harder. Even when a person experiencing estrogen dominance manages to motivate themselves to work out, their fatigue takes over. In this way, estrogen dominance can feel like a never-ending cycle that won't allow you to feel better and break through to the other side where you used to feel like "you."

One of the main signs of estrogen dominance is weight gain in the hips. Estrogen dominance can be the result of a variety of factors such as elevated body fat (which causes overproduction of estrogen), fluctuations in estrogen metabolization, or an imbalance in the estrogen-to-progesterone ratio (due to missed periods, irregular cycles, or menopause). Estrogen dominance worsens several conditions connected to estrogen, such as PCOS (polycystic ovarian syndrome), fibroids, endometriosis, and even breast and uterine cancers.

Simply put, estrogen dominance is pure hell.

Estrogen dominance occurs when estrogen levels are high relative to the other sex hormones, progesterone and testosterone. There is no definitive quantity of estrogen that results in estrogen dominance. It does, however, often occur during menopause.

Menopause brings a new set of challenges for most women, hormonal weight gain in particular. You may be scratching your head wondering why reduced estrogen levels would result in fat gain if estrogen is what makes women gain weight during puberty. Shouldn't estrogen levels similar to those before puberty result in less fat instead of more?

Here's what is happening: When you stop ovulating (due to menopause, a missed period, or an irregular cycle), your body does not experience the corresponding spike in progesterone that naturally occurs around day 14 of the menstrual cycle. As a result, estrogen levels are high relative to progesterone, creating estrogen dominance. With age, ovarian function begins to deteriorate, resulting in irregularity in the menstrual cycle, which throws off the natural balance of hormones in women. As much as we hate our period, it actually allows our hormones to rebalance and keeps our bodies from accumulating excess estrogen, which results in fat gain.

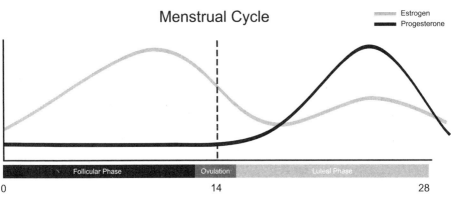

© Levi Bunnell

After menopause, a woman's body likes to hold on to fat cells because they provide more of the estrogen it's been missing due to the natural decline in estrogen that occurs when ovulation stops. The fat cells will never produce as much estrogen as the ovaries once did. However, this new low level of estrogen in the body causes a metabolic shift in the way your fat is distributed. It no longer moves to the hips and thighs; instead it goes to the belly. Low levels of estrogen during this stage result in fat gain because, again, progesterone levels are too low. This hormone imbalance creates a perfect storm for estrogen dominance.

Those with an elevated risk for estrogen dominance need to use nutritional strategies that facilitate fat loss under these conditions. The first thing you *do not* want to do under these circumstances is to go on a very low-calorie diet with a caloric deficit of 500 calories or more for extended periods of time. If you eat too few calories, you will prevent your body from having the opportunity to obtain the nutrients it needs from dietary fats, protein, and fiber to detox the excess estrogens from the liver.

If you have estrogen dominance, you should not, I repeat, *should not*, make weight loss your first goal. Instead, your number one priority should be to balance the hormones. For you, this might entail lifestyle improvements such as cutting out alcohol, exercising regularly, eliminating processed foods, drinking water instead of sugary beverages, and switching to home-cooked meals instead of takeout.

Estrogen and progesterone have a mutually beneficial relationship. However, when they fall out of balance, the imbalance leads to weight gain and also may cause excruciating periods, bloating, and fibroids. In order to reverse estrogen dominance, it boils down to identifying the underlying nutritional deficiencies and addressing them one at a time.

COMMON CAUSES OF HORMONAL IMBALANCES

Here are some common causes of hormonal imbalances and things you can do to correct them.

1. Insufficient Dietary Fat Intake

Dietary fats support monthly ovulation, which boosts fertility.[15] [16] This makes them necessary to support hormone production, including progesterone. Think of dietary fat as Wi-Fi. You don't realize how well it's working until it's not there and your access to the internet, or ability to ovulate, shuts down. Think of quality Wi-Fi compared to spotty Wi-Fi as the difference between quality fats like avocado, olive oil, and fatty fish as opposed to fried foods and low-quality oils.

Every time you experience a missed period or an irregular cycle, your body misses the opportunity to dispel excess estrogen. Each month, women experience a rise in estrogen to help increase the probability of fertilization. In the two weeks prior to menstruation, the body is pumping the uterus with extra estrogen to pad the uterine lining to receive an egg. During ovulation, this drives up libido. When ovulation does not result in a fertilized egg, estrogen levels decline and the excess estrogen left behind is shed through the menstrual period, resetting the uterus for another attempt at fertilization next month.

Popular low-fat diets would lead you to believe that eating more fat leads to more body fat, but hormonal fat gain isn't caused by eating healthy fats.

In fact, the insulin released when you eat carbohydrates causes your body to store carbs as fatty acids. The only time dietary fat intake results in fat gain is when you eat fats with a lot of carbs. Combining foods like cake, ice cream, chips, fries, and pasta drenched in cream sauce makes it too easy to overeat and pack on the pounds.[17]

2. Insufficient Dietary Fiber Intake

In addition to increasing dietary fat intake, obtaining proper amounts of fiber and micronutrients is essential to bringing the body out of a state of estrogen dominance. Increased levels of dietary fiber support the natural elimination of excess estrogens through the liver. On average, adults in the U.S. get about 10 to 15 grams of fiber per day, whereas they should be getting closer to 25 to 30 grams from whole foods, excluding fiber supplementation. Dietary fiber comes from carbohydrates composed of insoluble and soluble fiber. Although there is no recommended daily amount for fiber, 70 to 75 percent of your dietary fiber intake should come from insoluble fiber (the type of fiber that alleviates constipation and supports normal bowel movements — think greens) with the balance coming from soluble fiber (think whole grains, apples, etc.).

3. Zinc Deficiency

In their efforts to balance the estrogen-to-progesterone ratio, scientists have found that zinc supports lower estrogen while promoting higher progesterone. Zinc is essential for men, as it keeps testosterone from converting to estrogen by blocking aromatase (the enzyme responsible for this exchange). Think of zinc as the personal assistant to the enzymes behind the scenes, making biochemical reactions happen! Foods that are high in this powerhouse mineral include oysters, beef, chicken, seeds, nuts, legumes, and mushrooms.

4. Vitamin C Deficiency

Vitamin C is the Jamie Foxx of vitamins. It's been in the spotlight for as long as we can remember, but it's just that good. Vitamin C, also known as ascorbic acid, promotes many different things, from collagen formation, wound healing, and immune system support, to reducing high blood pressure, and reducing the risk of heart disease, to name a few. This vitamin also aids the ovaries, supporting monthly ovulation. Experts have shown vitamin C doses of at least 750 milligrams per day increase progesterone levels.[18] Low levels of dietary vitamin C are common among women who miscarry and have preterm pregnancy.[19] [20] Foods high in vitamin C include cruciferous vegetables (Brussels sprouts, broccoli, cauliflower), leafy greens, tomatoes, strawberries, guavas, kiwi, and snow peas.

5. Magnesium Deficiency

Magnesium is a low-key rock star. Sure, it's not as famous as vitamin C, but trust that magnesium has a crucial role that you would miss if it wasn't around. Magnesium is a macromineral that the body needs in large quantities. About 30 percent of the general population is deficient in magnesium, and roughly 50 percent of people with heart disease have magnesium deficiency. This mineral helps eliminate estrogen through a detoxification process in the liver, which in turn allows the body to excrete estrogen via urine or a bowel movement.[21] Magnesium is in real whole foods such as dark chocolate, avocado, nuts, seeds, fatty fish, whole grains, spinach, quinoa, and legumes.

6. Overconsumption of Estrogen Disruptors and Hormone-Rich Foods

Rebalancing your hormones entails eliminating products that contain estrogen disruptors such as plastics, personal care products containing xenoestrogens, and any pesticide-treated produce from a country outside of the U.S., such as Mexico. Mexico permits growers to use highly toxic pesticides, 111 of which are banned in the United States and other parts of the world.

To correct this, you'll need to avoid these foods. This also means becoming aware of what foods introduce estrogens, such as nonorganic meat and dairy, which have high levels of estrogens from source animals. Steering clear of hormone-loaded foods does not require you to go on a plant-based nutrition protocol. There are plenty of quality sources of animal-based proteins that are pasture-raised, grass-fed, grain-free, and easily accessible.

Plant-based diets are not superior to animal-based ones in this case, as produce can be full of estrogens, depending on the type of pesticides the agricultural process uses. Pesticide exposure is a well-known hormone disruptor of female reproduction.[22] Pesticides are an unfortunate — yet often considered necessary evil — way to control insects and disease and to boost yield of mass-produced vegetation. The entire point of pesticides is to maximize the yield of crops by killing off anything that may compromise the ability of the plants to grow; the problem is that the very thing that helps kill off bugs and diseases can also have a negative effect when humans are exposed, specifically reproductive issues in women. Point being, it is popular advice to go plant-based to avoid hormone-loaded foods, when in reality you can experience the same issues from plants due to the types of pesticides used in farming practices. Choosing produce from farmers' markets and organically grown ingredients will always be the preferred option for produce, especially for women with hormonal issues.

Remember, it's not enough to just eat Pinterest-worthy meals filled with veggies to bring your hormones back into balance. Eating clean is a wonderful start, but it does not guarantee that your macronutrient ratios are healthy. You can be eating 100 percent organic, non-GMO foods but still be too high in carbs, too low in protein, and not getting the correct amounts of fat for your hormonal needs. You need to eat in a way that facilitates the biochemical oxidation of stored body fat.

When your hormones are balanced, you not only look better, but you feel better. One-size-fits-most nutrition protocols do not work. A bodybuilder-style plan for a man who has zero concern for the fat content required to support ovulation does not work for most women. Targeting the appropriate macronutrient ratios for your needs is *crucial*.

TESTOSTERONE

Testosterone, the primary sex hormone in men, is in charge of growing muscle and developing the male reproductive system. Unlike the changes that women experience in puberty, when they gain fat, the onset of higher testosterone levels in males during puberty actually makes them drop body fat and increase lean muscle mass.

Imagine going from New York to Los Angeles by car. Even with a few breaks, it would take less than a week. Now imagine going from New York to Los Angeles by plane. It only takes a few hours, right? This is equivalent to the difference that testosterone makes when it comes to fat loss between women and men. So why not just give testosterone to women? There is a time and place for testosterone therapy for women; however, fat loss is not it. Although it would help with gaining muscle and losing fat, it would also throw off the female hormones and result in the masculinizing of a woman (think unpleasant side effects like an enlarged clitoris, facial hair, reduced breast tissue, changes to the voice, and acne, to name a few).

Thriving testosterone levels in men not only facilitate the growth of lean muscle and keep body fat levels down, but testosterone also boosts virility in men, resulting in healthy sperm count and motility. For both men and women, problems regarding body fat occur when testosterone levels drop.[23] Low testosterone levels in men are less than 300 ng/dl, whereas in women the low level is less than 25 ng/dl. Even though it's not the primary sex hormone in women, it still plays a role in muscle growth and fat loss. Low levels of testosterone in men are strongly correlated to higher levels of adiposity. In fact, obese men actually have approximately 30 percent lower testosterone levels compared to healthy men.[24] Now because men have substantially lower levels of estrogen compared to women, when they gain weight, that fat will not go to the hips, thighs, and buttocks like in women; it will go to the stomach.

How We Burn Fat: A Crash Course

Body fat is hands down the most concentrated energy source of the entire human body. Once you understand why, you will understand why it's harder to lose fat.

First, it is crucial to grasp that food is more complex than just energy in the form of calories, because burning calories does *not* mean you are burning fat. Losing fat is more complicated than working out harder and eating less. Legitimate fat loss occurs when your body uses free fatty acids for fuel instead of glucose (human blood sugar). If cells need more energy after the glycogen stores have been depleted, the cells will switch to fatty acids for fuel, a process known as *lipolysis*.

Lipolysis is the process of breaking down triglycerides into glycerol and free fatty acids. In order to drop stored body fat, it is essential for triglycerides to break down into their building blocks to facilitate the oxidation of free fatty acids. Because of its molecular structure, fat is harder to break down than carbs or protein. The amount of energy needed to oxidize each macronutrient is easiest to understand through the lens of the oxygen-to-carbon ratio. When a higher proportion of oxygen is present in the macromolecule, it is easier for oxidation to occur. It's not about the total oxygen content, but it is the ratio of carbon atoms to oxygen atoms that dictates the degree of how easily oxidation will occur. See the drawings on page 44 of basic protein, carbohydrate, and fat molecules.

When a fat molecule oxidizes, the reaction consumes oxygen and transforms into carbon dioxide (CO_2) and water (H_2O). This occurs when a sufficient level of oxygen is present to support oxidation, and glycogen is depleted, in order for the body to burn stored fat for fuel.

From a survival standpoint, the body does not want to part with stored body fat. The body evolved to anticipate periods of food scarcity, and stored body fat was the body's way of protecting itself.

The body must burn through its excess glycogen before switching over to stored body fat. A high-carb diet will increase glycogen stores, whereas a lower-carb diet will reduce them.

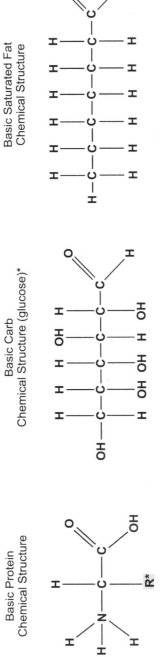

Basic Protein Chemical Structure

# of Carbon atoms = 2
# of Oxygen atoms = 2

Ratio of Carbon to Oxygen atoms:
1:1

R* Repeating amino acid chain sequence

Basic Carb Chemical Structure (glucose)*

# of Carbon atoms = 6
# of Oxygen atoms = 6

Ratio of Carbon to Oxygen atoms:
1:1

* = Glucose is typically a ring structure in water; however, for simplicity of demonstrating the carbon-to-oxygen ratio, it is being shown as a chain (it is found in this form about 0.02% of the time).

Basic Saturated Fat Chemical Structure

# of Carbon atoms = 7*
# of Oxygen atoms = 1

Ratio of Carbon to Oxygen atoms:
7:1

*Can be more carbons, depending on the type of fatty acid, increasing the ratio of carbon to oxygen

© Levi Bunnell

You can perform an hour of cardio every day and look pretty much the same, with no notable change in body fat. This is because burning calories does not necessarily mean your body is using adipose tissue as your fuel source. For this reason, it is essential to understand the role of each macronutrient in the body, what foods to get them from, and how much you need to consume of each to support your goals. (See Chapter 9 for more information on weight training, cardio exercise, and carb intake.)

When you are performing any form of physical activity, whether it's walking to your mailbox or going on a run, the first source of energy the body utilizes for fuel is carbohydrates in the form of glucose. The body is able to convert glucose in your cells or bloodstream to usable energy very quickly. For the body to use fat for energy, there must be an energy requirement that readily available resources such as glucose are not satisfying. Think of carbs as cash in a checking account and fats as funds in a savings account. Before you go through all the hassle of making a transfer or withdrawal from a savings account, you will use your liquid funds from a checking account first. When it comes to fat loss, the body does the same thing and uses available energy in the form of carbs first before tapping into fat stores.

A lot of clients come to me hoping to reduce fat in one specific area. Unfortunately, spot reduction doesn't work. Where your body pulls excess fat storage from first is going to depend on where it is most readily available. It also depends on your body type, genetics, and where you gained fat most recently. For example, you may want to lose fat just in your stomach, but if your most recent fat gain was in your limbs and chest, that is where your body will pull from first, the region where it has the easiest access.

Fat loss is a complex process that requires an excess of oxygen to oxidize a fatty acid. The body will take fat from the places that it can most readily metabolize it first, which tend to be the stomach, hips, glutes, and breasts. While it is not possible to spot-reduce body fat, you *can* focus on training specific muscle groups to add muscle in certain places. However, if body fat covers all of that muscle, you won't be able to see it.

. . .

Now that you have a basic understanding about fat — where we store it, why we store it, and how we burn it — it's time to talk about the next crucial piece of this puzzle: how your food influences fat loss.

3

How Macros Influence Fat Loss

The main reason most people do not look the way they want to is that they are not consuming the correct balance of macronutrients they need to biochemically alter their physique. True fat loss is more complex than burning calories. As you learned in Chapter 2, not only are there different types of fat, but there are also different forces that promote fat storage, which a person must reverse-engineer for successful fat loss. Changing your body composition is not as simple as eating less; there are many other challenges related to fat loss. The good news is that for every fat-loss problem, there is a corresponding nutritional strategy to overcome it.

When most people approach fat loss, they come with the "eating less is better" mentality, which is really the perspective of managed starvation. This is misguided and leads many people to eat too little, which then leaves them wondering why they don't feel good and can't function. Fat loss is about making wise choices about what is essential and what's nonessential. You can't just cut calories and expect to lower body fat. Some of those calories are providing essential nutrients that you cannot live without.

Weight loss is "easy," in that it's not hard to make the scale show a lower weight. However, the weight you are losing may only be water weight — or worse, lost muscle mass — leaving you with excess fat in spite of a lower weight. It's important for you to understand the foods you need to consume in essential quantities just to *function* before you can even start eliminating things to support fat loss. Too many people rush this process, asking, "How fast?" Instead, they should start by identifying their nutrient deficiencies, taking an "add to the plate" approach as opposed to "take away from the plate."

This chapter will demonstrate how each macronutrient impacts fat loss and begin to point you in the direction of the most appropriate approach for your personal circumstances. Basically, your body needs to be at a point biochemically where it prefers to oxidize stored body fat for energy. Fortunately, there is more than one way to do this. Thank goodness for science!

UNLOCKING YOUR MACRO TYPE: REAL STORIES, REAL SUCCESSES

Keeva, Protein-Fueled/Low-Carb Macro Type

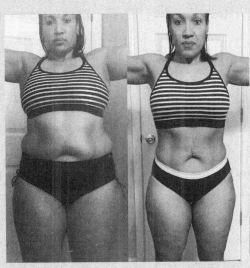

© Keeva Hamilton

Before   *After*

Keeva is a classic endomorph body type who struggles to drop body fat and gains it very easily. When we first started working together, she had high A1C levels, high cholesterol, thyroid issues, and was going through menopause. On top of that, she had a variety of food intolerances including dairy, gluten, and specific vegetables like broccoli, cauliflower, and Brussels sprouts. Because of her thyroid issues and cholesterol levels, a keto approach wasn't appropriate, so we needed to dial in her macros without going too low in carbs. During our time together, 5-foot, 3-inch Keeva went from over 230 pounds to around 150. She experienced a lifestyle overhaul, going from over 35 inches in her waist to 27. In her late 40s, she is now the leanest and healthiest she has ever been in her entire adult life. Macros gave Keeva her life back, and she inspires everyone with her can't-stop-won't-stop attitude. She shows up, she stays consistent, and she is the real deal when it comes to putting in the hard work. Other diet plans never worked for her, and she's thrived on this approach because it accounted for her specific carb tolerance level, her hormonal issues, and her thyroid issues.

Most people have a hard time making proper nutrition choices because they lack a fundamental understanding of the macronutrient composition of foods and how their body utilizes those macros. The big takeaway here is that you cannot compete with what you eat. I repeat: *You cannot compete with what you eat.* Far too many people underestimate how much food they actually eat and overestimate how much activity they get. If you believe you are active and eating healthy, yet you are not reaching your health goals no matter how much you try to eat right or how much you work out, chances are you have not tracked and measured your food portions. This does not mean that you need to take an obsessive approach to your nutrition, but it does mean that you will need greater mindfulness to reach your health goals. Portion control is the best place to begin.

The fuel available in fat, protein, and carbohydrates each have different biological influences on satiety, energy levels, metabolism, brain function, blood sugar, and how your body stores fat. Consuming the correct number of calories but the wrong ratios of protein, carbs, and fat is often the difference between feeling frustrated, tired, and stuck in a body you feel awful walking around in and feeling strong, energetic, and reaching your physique goals.

If you want to reduce body fat and increase lean muscle definition, you will need to rethink how you fuel your body. This is why macros matter. Your body *composition* will not shift to lower body fat while maintaining lean muscle if you aren't strategic about tailoring your nutrition to specific ratios.

When you have a specific, time-sensitive goal for your physique, fueling up with dialed-in macronutrient ratios is the best way to provide your body with what it needs. When you are trying to change your body fat percentage, lean muscle mass, and overall size and shape, you cannot expect arbitrary changes like "eating less carbs" or the ever so popular "trying to eat healthier" to achieve measurable progress.

Whether you realize it or not, you are already consuming a specific amount of protein, carbs, and fat every day. Chances are you haven't taken an in-depth look at what you are eating — and what you don't measure, you can't improve.

Auditing your current eating habits is the first step toward improving them. This may be a bigger wake-up call than you expect at first, because most people tend to underestimate how much they are eating. Every lick, bite, snack, drink, condiment — every single thing you consume in a day — *counts*. Even if a person eats only healthy, whole foods, they can still be overindulging in carbs and fats and not eating enough proteins. It's no surprise that most people do not count and measure their food portions. The average person eats when they are hungry, when they crave something specific, and only stop eating when they have eaten to a level of *emotional* satisfaction, usually well beyond their sense of *actual fullness*.

Your emotions are not a reliable gauge of how to eat. Specific macronutrient ratios for your body are. Let's dig deeper into each macronutrient to uncover the unique properties of each as it relates to fat loss.

Carbs: You Need Them

Carbohydrates are the most misunderstood food group when it comes to proper nutrition. They are typically the first to go when people begin a fat-loss program. I cringe when I hear people say, "Carbs are bad." No one should look at any macronutrient as good or bad but rather from the perspective of how their body will utilize it on a biochemical level and in what form it delivers vital nutrients to the body. Most people don't realize you can consume carbohydrates without gaining body fat if you select appropriate portions for your goals and make wise choices from the various dietary sources of carbohydrates.

Your relationship with carbohydrates plays a huge role in whether or not you will be able to drop fat following a conventional low-fat, higher-carb diet plan. Why? Some individuals are not able to functionally metabolize carbohydrates, meaning they have a lower carb tolerance. The good news is that if this is the case, your carb tolerance levels can be increased with improved nutrition over time. Your body needs to burn through carbs first before it can use stored body fat as fuel.

Carbohydrates are the first responders to the body's energy demands. Whenever you need energy, your body will first utilize glucose as its primary fuel source. When the body has depleted its carbs, it will switch to using fat as a fuel source. In addition, carbs are useful for promoting muscle growth and help replenish glycogen-depleted muscles.

So, what happens when you don't get enough carbs? Sounds impossible right? Who doesn't love carbs enough to eat the minimum amount? Believe it or not, not consuming sufficient carbs is a problem for some, and it directly impedes fat loss.

YOU NEED ENOUGH CARBS FOR FAT LOSS

When you aren't eating enough carbohydrates, your body goes into a catabolic state. This comes as a result of an extreme caloric deficit, which may be intentional due to extreme dieting, or unintentional, as your appetite may be naturally low or you may forget to eat. When this state occurs, *your body will seek to minimize muscle mass.* Not fat mass, mind you, because muscle mass takes more energy to maintain than body fat. If you under-fuel your body for extended periods of time, the first thing your body will part with is muscle, not fat. This also means that you can experience weight loss in a catabolic state, but since the quality of the weight you're losing is muscle and not fat, you won't experience the results you hoped for.

You can imagine the shock of my clients who come to me in this situation when I explain to them that they need to eat more carbohydrates, not less. I've had female ectomorph clients with high body fat, low muscle mass, and very high metabolic rates who have been eating less than 100 grams of carbs per day. By increasing their carb intake with quality carbohydrates to 200 to 300 grams per day, with some reaching as high as 400 to 500 grams, I've been able to help them drop their body fat. If you perpetually under-fuel your body, not getting enough carbs slows your progress.

Another circumstance where insufficient carb intake slows fat loss is when it interferes with your leptin levels. The leptin hormone, as we learned in Chapter 2, has two fundamental roles:

1. It sends the signal to your brain that you are full, lowering your appetite.
2. It lowers your metabolism when it perceives that your fat levels are getting too low (even though you may not be at your desired level of leanness yet).

When going low-carb, most people tend to drop calories at the same time. Over time, weight loss slows because the body is perceiving a reduction in available energy, which tends to boost hunger. If you are on a low-carb plan and you begin to experience a nagging sense of hunger that is not related to dehydration or your monthly cycle, this means your leptin levels are dropping and your body is getting the message, "Hello! Energy is becoming scarce; it's time to eat again!"

Too many nutritional strategies suggest that extreme caloric deficits are the answer to weight loss, but that only works to a certain point and results are short-term. Over time, your metabolism slows down due to low leptin levels, and this puts a hold on your ability to oxidize fat for fuel. The best way to work around this is a cycle of refeeding days where you elevate your carb intake on a training day. A refeed day is when you strategically increase your carb intake once a week to prevent fat-loss plateaus due to going too low in carbs for prolonged periods of time (longer than twelve weeks). This causes leptin levels to elevate, thereby sending the signal to your body that energy is no longer scarce and it is okay to increase energy expenditure, resulting in a higher metabolic rate.

TOO MANY CARBS CAUSE FAT GAIN

The body relies on dietary carbohydrates for energy in the same way cars rely on gasoline. Eating carbohydrates becomes problematic only when the body isn't utilizing them. Like putting gasoline in your car when the tank is already full, when we overeat carbs, the "spillover" fuel that we don't need gets stored as body fat. The body first uses carbs as energy for day-to-day activities and workouts. What it doesn't burn it stores as glycogen in the muscle cells, after it has depleted intramuscular glycogen during high-intensity exercise or resistance training. The muscle cells can store roughly 400 to 500 grams of carbs.

Once the muscle cells are "full," the next place the body holds carbs in the form of glycogen is the liver, which holds about 100 grams of carbs. The blood stores a very small amount of carbs as glucose; this value is very low, however, and we consider it insignificant as the body is always working overtime to move glucose out of the blood.

When the muscles and liver are "full" of carbs, the body converts the excess glucose into triglycerides and stores it as body fat. This is especially true when consuming carbs high on the glycemic index scale (high in sugar, low in fiber), because this results in a rapid spike in blood sugar, initiating the process of fat storage. This effect is stronger if you are already past the spillover point. Keep in mind that highly refined carbs, like the sugar in cakes, cookies, and ice cream, are easy to eat in excess as they don't boost your satiety in the same way as proteins and high-fiber carbs like vegetables or whole grains.

INSULIN RESISTANCE: A CYCLE OF HUNGER AND WEIGHT GAIN

Those who have insulin resistance face an added layer of complications that lead to fat gain. If you have ever felt like you are still hungry even though you just ate a carb-rich meal and wondered why you can't control yourself, it's not you. It's your body's inability to manage insulin.

This is because it's not your stomach that needs to use those carbs, it's your *cells!* If those cells can't access the energy available in carbohydrates, you will experience increased hunger even though you just ate. Your cells are telling your brain, "Hello! We're hungry. We need you to send some food over here!" and your brain gets the signal that you need to eat more.

This is what happens when you're *insulin-resistant*. Insulin, the messenger hormone, "escorts" carbs from the blood into the cells. If your cells are resistant to insulin, it means that insulin is knocking on the door to escort a glucose molecule inside, but instead of opening the door to let the glucose in, your cells ignore the knocking on the door. Your body then releases even more insulin from the pancreas to try to knock down the doors of your stubborn cells so you can get the energy you need to function. When that doesn't happen, your body makes you experience even more hunger. The cells are not able to obtain energy from the carbs, leaving your body starving on the cellular level.

If you're insulin-resistant or your energy needs are low because you are inactive, guess what? You are going to gain fat. If you have a healthy glucose metabolism, it only takes a small amount of insulin for the body to lower your body sugar. If your glucose metabolism is abnormal, your body will release more and more insulin. The pancreas is responsible for making insulin; however, it is also responsible for creating a fat-burning hormone called glucagon. When the pancreas is too busy producing insulin to shuttle glucose out of the blood and into the cells, it cannot focus on releasing this fat-burning hormone, and therefore you cannot be in a fat-burning state when you have insulin management issues. Intermittent fasting (limiting your eating window to 8 to 10 hours a day to put your body in an extended fasted state) can work well for those with insulin resistance, because it reduces the frequency of insulin spikes and allows an extended time for the pancreas to release glucagon to boost fat loss. You still need to be in a caloric deficit and eat according to your macro type, but by minimizing your insulin spikes, you can boost fat loss more readily.

UNLOCKING YOUR MACRO TYPE: REAL STORIES, REAL SUCCESSES

Breanna, Fat-Fueled/Low-Carb Macro Type

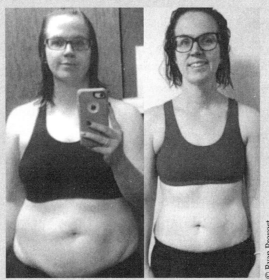

Before   *After*

Breanna has a very low carb-tolerance level and was able to lose over 33 pounds on a ketogenic protocol. Thanks to the macro-type approach, she was able to truly understand the appropriate portions for her specific goals, never felt hungry, reduced sugar cravings, and eventually learned how to experiment with macros and recipes, giving her the ultimate sense of freedom with her food. While her physical transformation was beyond impressive, the real transformation was her mental one. Her newfound knowledge has been priceless: She now knows and understands the science behind how to eat right for her body and recognizes that no food is good or bad and that it all can and should be had in moderation. Her ability to navigate a healthy relationship with food has led her to a sustainable healthy lifestyle.

Protein: You Need Enough, or You Can't Lose Fat

If you want a tight, toned, and lean physique, consuming the correct amount of protein is necessary to support those goals. Protein is essential for repairing damaged muscle fibers, burning fat, serving as the structure for skin, and maintaining properly functioning organs. In addition, protein is the precursor for enzymes, hormone production, immune function, and energy production.

In my own fat-loss journey, increasing protein levels was the game-changing piece of the puzzle. I'd tried every low-calorie diet under the sun. I was always able to lose weight, but I was never successful at losing *fat* until I got enough protein. For almost two decades, I believed that to get six-pack abs I needed to do tons of sit-ups, lots of cardio, and follow a very limited, low-calorie diet. But when I finally did achieve a six-pack, guess what? I hadn't performed a single sit-up, and I was only doing cardio three to five sessions a week. But my nutrition had been 100 percent spot-on for three to six months, and I was doing resistance training four times a week. Protein was the dominant macro that I needed to tweak to change my ability to lose body fat. I felt such a profound difference — as if I discovered the holy grail of fat loss — that I felt morally obligated to share my experience and the science behind it with anyone who struggled the same way I had. Learning the true value of protein and its role in nutrition literally changed my life.

What exactly is protein? The word *protein* refers to a type of molecule in food that breaks down into amino acids. Proteins are macromolecules consisting of long chains of amino acid subunits. There are two categories of amino acids: essential and nonessential. The body cannot make essential amino acids and must obtain them from food (examples are lysine and tryptophan), whereas it can produce nonessential amino acids (such as glutamine), so you don't necessarily need to get these from food. Unfortunately, most people do not obtain sufficient levels of protein from whole foods.

Why is protein so important when it comes to fat loss? Protein is the nutrient that builds the body and enables you to change your body composition to drop body fat without losing muscle mass. Protein is the only macronutrient that contains nitrogen, which in the right amounts forces your body to use fat as a fuel source. When the body uses fat for fuel, it prevents the body from going into a catabolic state in which it breaks down muscle tissue to obtain the amino acids it needs. Burning fat for fuel also makes it easier to shed excess fat and decreases appetite — a win-win.

The body requires a positive balance of nitrogen to switch over to lipolysis, the biological process where you burn fat for fuel. When you consume enough dietary protein to boost your nitrogen content, it's easier for your body to lose fat while sparing lean muscle tissue.

This seems simple enough, but it's easy to get confused by marketing. Food companies market a lot of "health foods" as good sources of protein. But just because a food has protein doesn't mean it's a good source of protein. For example, almonds contain protein, but 1 ounce of almonds only contains 6 grams of protein, 6 grams of carbohydrates, and 14 grams of fat. From a macronutrient perspective, this food is 77 percent fat.

This is why the macronutrient approach can give you a true edge when it comes to changing your physique: When you only pay attention to calories, not macronutrients, it is easy to miss the ideal range for your specific goals. Tracking protein content on a daily basis is essential when you want to reduce body fat and gain or maintain lean muscle mass. In order to add lean muscle tissue, you need to consume more protein than your body requires for its basic daily functions (DNA replication, metabolic processes, normal growth, cell replacement, muscle tissue repair, and so on).

If you don't eat enough protein to sustain your body's needs, you may lose weight but not gain or maintain muscle. This is why it's important to remember that fat loss and weight loss do not necessarily go hand in hand. If you restrict calories but don't eat enough protein, your body will cannibalize its own muscle tissue to secure the necessary amino acids to function — that's *catabolism*. This is why you can lose weight but not lose fat or inches and why I do not recommend gauging your progress based on the number on the scale. You might be dropping weight but losing muscle, or you could be gaining weight while losing fat. That's why it's far better to use body measurements, improvements in energy, and photos to track your progress. You need to create a positive nitrogen balance — by eating enough protein — to prevent catabolism and maintain your tight lean muscles, which will make it easier to drop the unwanted fluff.

Insufficient protein intake can also impede fat loss if you are overtraining. You can have too much of a good thing, exercise included. Intense resistance training breaks down muscle tissue. Muscle growth occurs when these tissues have time to recover and receive enough dietary protein to support regeneration. Too much training in conjunction with a shortage of protein leaves you with a negative nitrogen balance.

After an intense session of resistance training, the body is able to absorb nutrients like a sponge. Timing training sessions too close together can result in an insufficient supply of nutrients to support sustained growth. While fitness is important to overall health, it is crucial to remember that exercise is a form of stress on the body. In the right amounts, this type of stress is appropriate to support fat loss. However, excessive stress and overtraining can be taxing not only on the muscles but also the organs and brain, and it can inhibit the body's ability to retain vitamins and minerals. Ironically, excessive training can dramatically reduce your physical performance if you've exhausted your body's stores of vitamins and minerals. The fix: protein supplementation and recalculating the body's total daily energy expenditure (TDEE), as I'll demonstrate in Chapter 6.

THERE IS SUCH A THING AS TOO MUCH PROTEIN

It's highly unlikely that you will overshoot your protein intake on a high-protein nutrition plan when protein is more than 35 percent of your total calorie budget. It's challenging to hit protein macros that high, so you might struggle to some extent to hit these values.

But on the ketogenic diet, a fat-dominant approach with modest protein levels and very low carb content, you need to watch your protein intake. While it's generally a good thing to increase your protein content, that goes against the logic of nutritional ketosis. When your body is utilizing fat for fuel, carb content needs to be very low to minimize insulin spikes. But people with insulin resistance are more likely to experience a spike in insulin *after consuming high levels of protein,* to the point where it can actually kick you out of nutritional ketosis.

This happens because protein can break down into carbs through the chemical reaction known as *gluconeogenesis* (GNG).[1] This occurs when the body creates glucose from the non-carb macros such as proteins. GNG isn't necessarily a bad thing; it means the body is naturally creating the glucose it needs to fuel parts of the bodily tissues that are not responsive to ketones. But it means you need to carefully calculate your protein intake on the ketogenic diet if you are a Fat-Fueled Macro Type (as described in detail in Chapter 5).

Fats: You Need to Eat Fat to Burn Fat

Fats are the most energy-dense macronutrient, containing more than twice as many calories per gram as proteins and carbs. For a long time, we were taught to fear fat because of its higher calorie count. But you can and should consume fats as part of your daily food intake. Consuming dietary fat slows down blood sugar spikes and slows the rate at which your body stores excess sugar (glucose) as body fat.

There is a lot of confusion and conflicting information surrounding fat intake. Despite the fact that the USDA recommends a low-fat, high-carb nutrition approach, this approach *does not work* for most people. Throughout the 1970s, '80s, '90s, and early 2000s, aka the era of low-fat dieting, we were told that cutting fat from our diet was the best way to avoid chronic illnesses (such as obesity, diabetes, heart disease). This led to an entirely new low-fat/nonfat food industry with products like nonfat milk and low-fat potato chips. It also attached a new stigma to fatty foods like bacon, butter, chicken skin, and steak. We were led to believe that these foods were not only bad for our hearts but would make us fat. Manufacturers compounded the problem even further by reducing fat content to create "low-fat" versions of processed foods — remember low-fat and supposedly "guilt-free" cookies? The problem is, these processed foods substituted the fat with refined carbohydrates, which trigger insulin production, making it (ironically) harder to lose fat.

The idea that "fat is bad" is based on outdated studies from the 1950s that imply a correlation between heart disease and saturated fat intake.[2] Scientists based this theory on a study of subjects in specific countries (Japan, Italy, the U.K., Canada, Australia, and the U.S.) that had both higher levels of saturated fat intake and higher rates of heart disease. What most people did not realize is that the scientists reporting this study conveniently ignored data that was available from sixteen other countries that did not support their theory. When a different group of scientists accounted for all of the available data from a total of twenty-two countries, their conclusion was the opposite. They found that those who consumed the highest percentage of saturated fat had the *lowest* risk of heart disease.

Since the early 2000s, research has slowly shown the errors in the "all fat is bad" argument. But the damage of misinformation goes on. As a result, many people have had nutrient deficiencies due to insufficient fat intake coupled with excess intake of refined carbs, which they haven't been able to address.

Today we understand that fats are necessary parts of a healthy lifestyle and body. The reality is, consuming dietary fat does not activate the hormonal triggers that initiate the storage of body fat. Consuming carbs, on the other hand, activates insulin, the fat-storing hormone.

Depending on one's macro type, some people need to consume more fats than other macronutrients. Throughout history, from the Paleolithic era all the way to modern Atkins and keto-style nutrition programs, humans have utilized fat as a fuel source. The keto diet works by lowering your carb intake while raising your fat intake, forcing your body to use fat for fuel. This makes it easier to burn through stored body fat as energy because your body doesn't need to burn through carbs first. Under these circumstances, when your body senses that it needs energy, it can pull energy from your stored fat because it's in a state of nutritional ketosis. Scientists first developed the keto diet to manage epilepsy but have since recognized its potential to mitigate the negative health issues associated with excess insulin.[3]

When you consume healthy fats, your body converts these fats into ketones in the liver, which it can use as fuel. To put this in macronutrient terms, the keto diet is high in fat, moderate in protein, and very low in carbs. This breaks down to 70 to 75 percent fat, 20 to 25 percent protein, and only 5 percent carbs. Most people first react to these ratios with alarm, saying, "How am I going to live on 5 percent carbs? That's like a single cracker in a day!"

That's one way to look at it, but the keto diet offers an opportunity to look at carbs differently. If you only think about the carbs you are used to consuming in excess, the idea of taking them away may sound like a recipe for starvation. Instead of thinking of refined carbs like crackers, which will cause you to go over 5 percent carbs very quickly, think of high-volume nutrient-dense carbs like kale, spinach, arugula, Brussels sprouts, cauliflower, broccoli, mushrooms, blueberries, and raspberries, which are substantially lower in carbs and higher in fiber, enabling you to consume more food volume by shifting the type of carbs you consume.

TOO MUCH FAT WILL STALL FAT LOSS

Most of my clients and followers make the same mistake when it comes to weight loss: They eat too much fat coupled with refined, processed carbs. Before you scratch your head and say, "Wait, I thought you just said fats are good and I need them?" let me stop you. Fats are good, they have many wonderful properties and benefits, not to mention they make food taste amazing. As usual, the issue is context.

Let's start with the standard American diet — aka "the eat 'whatever' approach." If you aren't intentional about how you select your foods, you will end up eating the most readily available foods, which tend to be high-fat, low-protein, and have lots of refined carbs. I'm talking about fast food, pasta, croissants, donuts, cookies, baked goods, cheesecake, milkshakes, fries, chips, crackers, granola bars, candy, movie theater popcorn, and any combination of ingredients that are high in fat and high in carbs.

As you can see, it's not hard to find high-fat, high-carb foods. They taste good, they're cheap, they provide a temporary sense of comfort (think comfort foods), and you don't have to travel far to get them. If you find yourself defaulting to these foods, you are setting yourself up for failure. You can achieve fat loss by going high in protein, low in fat, and moderate in carbs. You can also achieve fat loss by going high in fat, low in carbs, and moderate in protein. **But you cannot achieve fat loss by going high in fat and high in carbs at the same time.**

There are a few problems that make a high-fat and high-carb diet a disaster when it comes to fat loss. This eating style is usually low in protein, which keeps your body from being in a positive nitrogen balance, which it needs to use fat for fuel. You will also experience high insulin and blood sugar levels, making it almost impossible to burn through your glycogen to the point where you can tap into stored fat for fuel. When your blood sugar is always elevated and you are eating *often,* you trigger your hormones to store fat.

The addictive nature of high-carb, high-fat food puts your body in a perfect storm of perpetual fat gain. Each time you eat these foods, you spike your insulin, which drives your cravings up and makes you eat more, instead of settling your hormones with higher levels of protein and fiber.

· · ·

Now that you have a baseline understanding of macros, we're going to look at carb tolerance and help you determine whether you need a lower, moderate, or higher carb diet — the results might surprise you!

4

Discover Your Carb Tolerance

B efore you even read this chapter, you might worry that I'm going to tell you that you need to part ways with carbs. Before jumping to conclusions, remember: Carbs are not the enemy. I know that this might sound contrary to what you've heard. If you're like most of my clients, you've spent hours scouring the internet for information on which carbs are safe to eat and in what amounts — only to find conflicting answers, most of which aren't based on actual *science*. I get it. You want real answers. You are sick and tired of the disappointing advice of your colleague, friend, or family member who raves about the diets that helped them lose a hundred pounds, only to find their plan doesn't work for you.

By the time many clients find me, they have tried program after program and have found it impossible to get results or even sustain a highly restrictive plan that doesn't work in the real world. When you learn about your macro type in the next chapter, you'll be able to conceptualize what an ideal diet looks like for you (not your mother, sister, or best friend). But before you start counting macros, it is crucial to understand the key variable that makes shedding unhealthy levels of stored body fat so challenging for some: carb tolerance.

In 2015, I started working with a client named Leann. She appeared to be healthy physically, but her years-long struggle with dieting and weight loss had distorted her body image. So much so, in fact, that during our first two consultations, she wouldn't even tell me her weight. She had deep negative associations with the number on the scale and found it better for her sanity to not weigh herself. After reviewing her baseline photos and body measurements, I estimated that she was between 30 and 35 percent body fat and had a maximum of 25 pounds to lose. Even a solid 10- to 15-pound reduction would be more than enough to get her to a place where she could feel better about her physique.

Leann had been adhering to a paleo lifestyle and was a big-time foodie. She always ate the highest-quality ingredients and loved cooking delicious, Pinterest-worthy meals. People often tout the paleo diet as the best method for fat loss due to its high restrictions on carbs. But unbeknownst to her, Leann's paleo diet was far too low in carbs for her macro type. When we began working together, she had a lot of carb confusion.

The intention of the paleo lifestyle is to focus on eating unprocessed whole foods while avoiding inflammatory foods like gluten, dairy, soy, legumes, grains, and processed or artificial sugars. Leann ate lots of healthy fats, moderate to moderately low proteins, and moderately low carbs. She didn't bother keeping track of calories, and she never considered her macros. In two years of following a paleo lifestyle, Leann didn't lose any body fat. In fact, she'd gained a little weight.

The first thing we had to do was determine her daily caloric intake. Even though the foods she ate were all healthy and organic, we discovered that she was eating upwards of 3,000 calories a day while leading a relatively sedentary lifestyle. Leann was floored to learn she was eating that much. The second issue was that Leann was eating a high-fat diet that didn't match her macro-type needs. Lastly and most importantly, Leann was eating far too few carbs. Her intake was less than 40 to 50 grams per day, when she could afford to consume upwards of 150 grams with ease. It blew Leann's mind to learn that she could eat over 150 grams of carbs a day and still drop body fat. Once we matched Leann's macro type with her carb tolerance level, she experienced a breakthrough in her progress. In twelve weeks, she was able to drop 4 inches from her waist while consuming over 1,700 calories a day. She slid into clothes that had been too tight for over five years.

In this chapter, we will uncover the factors that contribute to your personal carb tolerance, the same piece of information that pushed Leann past her fat-loss plateau. Armed with this knowledge, you'll be able to set the balance of your macronutrients within your macro type and ensure your carb intake is optimal for your goals.

Carb tolerance is a measure of the optimal amount of carbohydrates your body can process on a biochemical level. On one end of the spectrum, there are people who cannot process carbs without throwing their metabolism out of whack (i.e., prediabetics or diabetics). These folks need to go very low-carb. On the other end, there are those with very high carb tolerances who are naturally lean and struggle to gain muscle and weight. This leaves a wide range in between, which is where most people find themselves.

Carb tolerance sets the tone for your entire nutrition strategy. Over the past ten years of working with clients, I have found that evaluating how the body responds to carbohydrates forms the foundation for a successful nutrition protocol, in terms of both a plan's effectiveness and a person's ability to adhere to it. Your ideal macronutrient balance stems from this underlying bio-individual relationship between carbohydrates and your glucose metabolism, sex hormones, thyroid hormones, digestive enzymes, gut health, and activity level. The good news is, there is no right or wrong level — this is all about the right level of carbs for *your* body.

UNLOCKING YOUR MACRO TYPE: REAL STORIES, REAL SUCCESSES

Nina, Fat-Fueled Macro Type

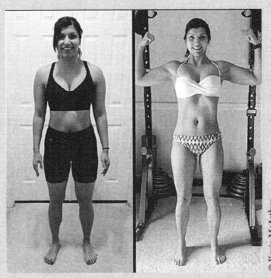

Before   *After*

When I first met Nina she didn't realize she had carb tolerance issues. She didn't have diabetes and was never diagnosed with a high A1C. She started out on a traditional high-protein, low-fat approach. But she experienced a breakthrough when we lowered her carbs and increased her fat intake. While she was not prediabetic and didn't have a concentrated amount of fat in the torso or lower body, she did have a family history of diabetes and experienced high fasting blood glucose values. As someone who struggled with weight for years and had tried highly restrictive, very low-calorie plans, she is thrilled to feel better than ever before and look the best she ever has in her adult life. She's at a healthy weight and has an improved relationship with food. She was 145 pounds when we started working together (after first topping the scales over 150 pounds before losing weight on her own). Once we started, she was able to drop 15 pounds and is now a healthy and sustainable 130 pounds at 5 feet, 6 inches. Since dialing in her nutrition, her insulin sensitivity has improved, meaning she can handle slightly higher carbs once in a while but feels best when she keeps them moderately low. Her waist was over 30 inches when we started and is now a lean 26 inches.

There are a number of factors that influence your personal carb tolerance. Let's take a closer look at them.

Your Metabolism Hormones

Insulin and glucagon are the two most important hormones responsible for regulating metabolism, blood sugar, and the other macromolecules (proteins and fats). Together, they engage in a process called *glucose homeostasis*, which means they help the body maintain the narrow window of blood glucose levels it requires for optimal function.

While several parts of the body can use either protein or fat as fuel, the brain and red blood cells can only use glucose. To achieve this balance, insulin supports the uptake of macromolecules, while glucagon supports the breakdown of macromolecules. In other words, insulin gathers resources to support your energy needs (which can drive fat gain) and glucagon spends that energy (which drives fat loss).

For our purpose of understanding fat loss, we only need to know how these hormones behave in two scenarios: when blood glucose is too low or too high. When your blood glucose is low, your body is in a state of hypoglycemia. When this happens, the pancreas will release glucagon because your body needs more sugar to return to glucose homeostasis. The glucagon hormone will then convert fats and amino acids (aka protein) into glucose in a process called *gluconeogenesis*. Through this process, glucagon makes energy from body fat, which can be a good thing. However, if this becomes an ongoing strategy, it begins to become an issue. Going too low in carbs for too long can make you feel weak, give you brain fog, and induce a general feeling of being "off."

Conversely, when glucose is too high, glucagon's sidekick, insulin, steps up and shuttles glucose out of the blood and into the cells. From there, the liver and muscle cells store the excess glucose via a process called *glycogenesis*. When the liver and muscles are at their capacity for glucose, the body will store these excess carbs as fat.

If you have been in a lifelong battle with body fat, you most likely have been throwing off your body's natural state of glucose homeostasis. In this chapter, we will break down the key factors that impact your bio-individual carb tolerance level so you can discover the most appropriate range of carbs you should consume for optimal fat loss and your body's needs. Then, I'll give you a quiz to help you figure out your carb tolerance.

Glucose Metabolism

Carbohydrates fuel cellular reactions. When you consume a carbohydrate, it breaks down in the blood into its simplest form, the glucose sugar molecule. The body then transports glucose to the cells to power physical activity. How easily your body can obtain cellular energy from carbohydrates determines the efficiency of your glucose metabolism. When your cells are not able to absorb energy from glucose, problems arise. This can be caused by a number of factors.

The first issue, as introduced in Chapter 3, is insulin resistance, which affects about one-third of the population of the United States.[1] Insulin is a vital hormone that has several regulating functions, one of which is lowering your blood sugar. When you experience a temporary spike in blood sugar, your pancreas releases insulin to move the glucose out of your blood and into your cells. If your cells are nonresponsive to insulin, three problems occur: First, your cells can't receive the energy they need. Second, even though you've eaten, you are starving on a cellular level, so your body continues to send you hunger signals. Third, your blood sugar rises (which is toxic to your system), resulting in fatigue and brain fog. Under these circumstances, as a protective measure, your body shuttles the excess glucose out of your blood and stores it as fat.

It can be hard to tell if you've experienced insulin resistance, although a persistent struggle with fat loss is a potential sign. If you aren't sure if this applies to you, consider these early symptoms and warning signs:

- Fasting glucose >100mg/dL
- HbA1C levels >5.7
- Blood pressure >130/80
- Waist >35 inches for women and >40 inches for men
- HDL cholesterol >50mg/dL in women and >40mg/dL in men

Some of these markers are determined in tests requested by your doctor in a routine physical, but not all of them. (If you have growing concerns or suspect you may have insulin resistance, I suggest you consult your doctor and request these tests.) Insulin resistance is a sign that your body is struggling to manage blood sugar and is best measured by testing your A1C levels via the blood test for HbA1C. If you are between 5.7 and 6.4, you are considered prediabetic. If you are over 6.5, you are considered diabetic.

Another factor that can affect your cells' ability to absorb carbs is the amount of carbs you consume. When I ask someone how their body responds to carbs, right away most people tell me they think they have a low carb tolerance because they tend to feel bloated after eating carbohydrates. News flash: Carbohydrates retain about 3 grams of water for every 1 gram of carbs you consume. This is one of several reasons the body prefers to store fat as energy and not carbs. The hydrophobic nature of fats enables the body to store them in a more condensed form than it can with hydrophilic carbs. So, if you just ate a restaurant-sized portion of pasta (say 100 grams of carbs) in a single sitting, it will cause you to retain about 300 grams of water. Of course, you'll feel bloated! This may have absolutely nothing to do with your carb tolerance level.

A true sign of carb tolerance issues is when you experience problems even when you eat modest portions of carbs. If you had pancakes for breakfast and feel tired before lunchtime or you experience fatigue, brain fog, bloating, and are hungry right after eating, then you likely have a true carb intolerance.

Even if you have a moderate or moderately low carb tolerance, that does not mean you need to be on a very low-carb nutrition plan such as the keto diet. Your optimal level of carbs may still be much higher than you realize, once you've balanced it with the correct levels of fiber, protein, and fat.

When it comes to restricting calories and carbs, I always encourage clients to resist the urge to make drastic changes to their overall intake unless absolutely necessary. For instance, if your lifestyle has been sedentary and most of your diet has been low-fiber, sugar-rich carbohydrates with lots of fats, making even modest reductions in carbs and eating carbs with more fiber and less sugar can not only initiate fat loss, but high-fiber carbs will help you feel fuller, so you're getting the results you want without feeling hungry. This counterintuitive experience is one of my favorite things to witness.

UNLOCKING YOUR MACRO TYPE: REAL STORIES, REAL SUCCESSES

Jacqueline, Fat-Fueled Macro Type

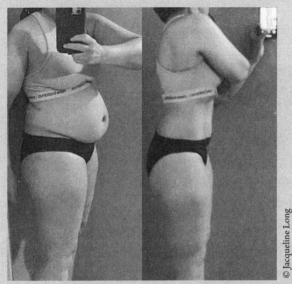

© Jacqueline Long

Before   *After*

Meet Jacqueline, one of my clients who has experienced a game-changing journey with her fat loss using a fat-dominant plan that's ideal for her low tolerance to carbs. She has lost 10 inches off her waist and about 20 pounds in just five months. In spite of her low carb tolerance, we were able to make two of her favorite higher-carb foods — mangoes and rice — fit into her macros! At 56 years old, Jacqueline is dealing with perimenopause and moving into menopause, so weight loss has become more of a challenge. We have been able to navigate those hurdles by increasing her fats and lowering her carbs, allowing her to drop weight in a consistent and sustainable way. She has been able to navigate the challenges of hormone imbalances with ease thanks to this eating plan!

Fat loss with a low carb tolerance is not always about eating less; it's about eating well. If you have a lower carb tolerance, you don't need to eliminate carbs from your life.

Sex Hormones

As we learned in Chapter 2, sex hormones play a huge role in the composition, distribution, and accumulation of stored body fat. So, what do sex hormones have to do with insulin and carb tolerance?

All of the body's hormones determine how the body deals with food. Insulin doesn't function in a vacuum. When your sex hormones are imbalanced, they introduce shifts in your mood, stress, metabolism, and digestion, among other functions. Sex hormones can become imbalanced, regardless of whether you are overweight, due to lifestyle factors such as chronic stress, poor quality of sleep, regular alcohol consumption, and eating too many refined carbohydrates. These take a toll on your body over time. If your sex hormones are off balance, you're not alone.

We tend to only think of the most extreme expressions of sex hormone imbalances. When estrogen is too high, we think of perimenopause or polycystic ovarian syndrome (PCOS). When estrogen is too low, we think of menopause. The same goes for men. When testosterone is too low, we think of erectile dysfunction and obesity. When testosterone is too high, we think of balding, aggressive mood swings, and excessive muscle growth. We are missing the broader context of how estrogen and testosterone interact with insulin and its ability to regulate blood glucose.

THE IMPACT OF LOW ESTROGEN ON CARB TOLERANCE

Estrogen is the most important hormone in females for regulating mood and reproductive health. Estrogen levels decline based on the time of the month, PCOS, or menopause. Lower estrogen levels can cause symptoms such as irregular periods, low fertility, poor sleep quality, vaginal dryness, urinary tract infections, and increased hunger.

Women of childbearing age can experience issues with their carb tolerance at different points in their menstrual cycle. Day 1 through day 14 of the menstrual cycle (day 1 being the onset of your period), called the *follicular phase,* designates the time between the start of a woman's period and the day she ovulates. During this time, estrogen levels are climbing to prepare the body to release an egg and the body is more sensitive to insulin. This is a good thing as it means resistance to insulin is down and the body has a higher carb tolerance. This is important to note for those of you who are very sensitive to carb intake, as you may want to time carb-rich meals for the first half of your cycle.

Once a woman ovulates (releases an egg that is primed for fertilization), her estrogen levels decline, and as a result her hunger rises. This marks the beginning of the second half of the menstrual cycle, called the *luteal phase.* This part of the cycle is when PMS sets in, and women experience corresponding surges in hunger.[2] This rise in hunger has two causes: First, the body is expending more energy due to hormonal shifts. Second, when estrogen levels drop, insulin resistance increases. Not only is the body burning more calories, but its ability to handle carbs is compromised. When this happens in a woman with an already low carb tolerance, it's best for her to manage cravings with increased dietary fats and proteins and with carbs that won't spike her insulin levels, such as veggies.

Low estrogen levels can also result from PCOS, by far the most prevalent endocrine disorder affecting women. PCOS can cause decreased fertility, excessive facial hair, irregular periods, and weight gain. Women with this condition tend to experience insulin resistance and higher testosterone levels. Compromised glucose tolerance levels occur in about two-thirds of women with PCOS.[3] This hormone imbalance drives the body to experience intense carb cravings. Ironically, even though your body craves carbs, it cannot process them due to hormone imbalances. Talk about a recipe for frustration! The good news is that by combining a lower-carb-tolerance nutrition strategy, lifestyle changes, and doctor-supervised medication, you can mediate this cycle of hormonal masochism.

UNLOCKING YOUR MACRO TYPE: REAL STORIES, REAL SUCCESSES

Kandis, Fat-Fueled/Low-Carb Macro Type

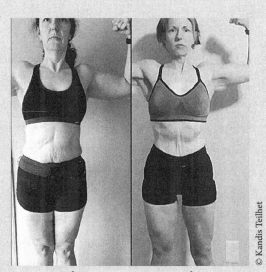

© Kandis Teilhet

Before   After

Kandis and I have worked together for over two years, navigating a wide range of health concerns, from hormone imbalances to fibromyalgia, and a variety of food intolerances. A mesomorph, she started with a much more moderate carb plan but has seen the greatest results when we've brought her carb levels down. Working with clients like Kandis, who don't fit the typical macros model, is what inspired me to write this book: She is living proof that carb tolerance is an important factor and can make or break the success of a plan. After some trial and error, we found she thrives on a ketogenic protocol when she is fueled by fats and not carbs. One of the biggest takeaways from Kandis's transformation is that it occurred in two phases. The first was her initial weight-loss effort to drop body fat; the next was her goal to increase her caloric intake and to add muscle mass, which we were able to do on keto. During her fat loss, her daily intake ranged from 1,400 to 1,750 calories. Now we have moved her from 1,400 calories to 2,600 at 5 feet, 8 inches and approximately 135 pounds. She is feeling stronger than ever before and is 50 years young. She is an example of someone who has sustained the ketogenic lifestyle and is in it for the long haul!

Another cause of low estrogen levels is menopause, both natural and surgical. Menopause is when a woman has gone twelve months without a menstrual cycle, marking the end of the body's monthly ovulation and fertility. The effects of menopause can also occur earlier in life if a woman undergoes ovary-removal surgery. During menopause, the body produces less estrogen and testosterone, resulting in low libido, hot flashes, weight gain, and mood swings. You would think the end of your period would be a walk in the park; menopause is anything but.

So, what does low estrogen have to do with insulin? When the sex hormones decline, it causes fluctuations in your blood sugar, resulting in erratic cravings. Blood sugar management is critical in navigating menopause and the years leading up to it. You can no longer make random food choices without considering their impact on your hormones. The resulting distress is not worth the temporary pleasure. Unlike in your childbearing years, 5 pounds of weight gain after a long weekend can trigger upwards of 25 pounds of additional weight gain in the following weeks and months. Menopause doesn't afford you the luxury of being able to get back on track with the same ease you had when you were younger.

When estrogen levels drop, the body becomes more resistant to insulin. This means the cells in the muscles, liver, and brain need more insulin per unit of glucose in the blood to shuttle that glucose into the cells. As a result, sugar spends more time in the blood, making it more likely that the body will store it as fat.

Eating with lowered estrogen levels requires mindful choices. Most people think they only gain fat when they eat foods that are obviously low in nutrient density, such as donuts or chips, but if you have low estrogen, even a breakfast of yogurt and oatmeal will trigger the hormones responsible for fat gain. Worse, if you have reached the point where you have accumulated an uncomfortable level of belly fat, your cravings may be even stronger because your body is sending loud and clear signals that it wants sugar! You aren't weak and you aren't crazy; you're just not managing your blood sugar.

THE IMPACT OF HIGH ESTROGEN ON CARB TOLERANCE

"High estrogen" tends to mean high relative to progesterone, aka estrogen dominance, which we learned about in Chapter 2. If left untreated, estrogen dominance can lead to breast and ovarian cancer. Irregular or missed periods can trigger estrogen dominance since the body doesn't receive the usual spike in progesterone that occurs after ovulation. Remember, not only do the ovaries produce estrogen, but so do the fat cells. If your body fat levels are creeping up, so will your estrogen levels.

Excess estrogen leads to health issues such as weight gain, abnormal bleeding, breast sensitivity and tenderness, fatigue, bloating, depression, and mood swings. In the case of estrogen dominance, a woman's first priority should always be to rebalance her estrogen levels before focusing on weight loss. When women jump the gun and focus on losing weight by lowering their calories, they end up eliminating vital nutrients they need to keep their hormones balanced, which makes for a vicious cycle. If you're estrogen dominant, instead of arbitrarily cutting calories and carbs, I recommend focusing on carb quality and quantity and being mindful to cut out all processed sugars, caffeine, and alcohol. This is not a ticket to eat all the carbs either; moderate to moderately low levels can work well in this case.

THE IMPACT OF LOW TESTOSTERONE ON CARB TOLERANCE

Testosterone levels are naturally lower in women than men, but women still need this hormone to maintain a healthy libido, generate new cells, and support the development of other hormones. When something compromises a woman's ovaries or adrenal glands, her testosterone levels drop below the healthy range. Testosterone levels can also drop when women partake in extreme caloric deficits for prolonged periods of time (along with muscle loss, another reason extreme dieting is not healthy or ideal). Doctors often misdiagnose low testosterone in women as stress or depression, which leaves women blaming themselves for an autonomous hormonal issue. For women with low testosterone, consuming a moderate amount of quality carbs is ideal and will support the body in bringing the hormones back into balance.

Testosterone is the primary sex hormone for men. They require much higher levels of testosterone to promote a healthy sex drive, maintain muscle, and support the body in metabolizing fat. According to the *Journal of Clinical Endocrinology,* men experience a 25 percent decline in testosterone within 2 hours of consuming 75 grams of sugar, regardless of whether they have pre-existing issues metabolizing glucose.[4] Even healthy men ages 20 to 39 experienced this abrupt drop in testosterone. To put this in perspective, a 12-ounce can of Red Bull contains 37 grams of sugar. Drinking just two cans of this sugary beverage can catalyze a series of reproductive health issues in men, including low testosterone and reduced sperm count. For men with low testosterone levels, it is common to experience reduced carb tolerance levels, increased body fat (visceral fat in particular), and increased insulin resistance.[5]

Before you write off carbs as testosterone killers, remember that this is specific to refined carbohydrates in large doses. One can maintain peak testosterone levels through a diet high in slow-digesting, low-sugar, high-fiber carbs. This includes complex carbs like vegetables, fruit, and whole grains.

UNLOCKING YOUR MACRO TYPE: REAL STORIES, REAL SUCCESSES

Justin, Protein-Fueled Macro Type

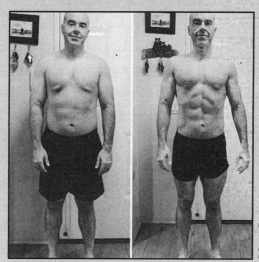

Before   *After*

© Justin Best

Meet Justin, who came to me wanting to get lean and muscular at the same time. He was familiar with the gym and running but was missing pieces to put it together to see the results he truly wanted. The biggest change was actually eating more than he thought he needed. He went from 212 to 184 pounds. During this time, he dropped his waist from 35 to 28.5 inches while reshaping his 41-inch chest and back. He needed high protein, low fat, and moderate carbs. He experienced no major issues to progress once he was dialed in with his macros aligned for a protein-fueled approach to his nutrition. His calories ranged between 1,900 and 2,400 during this shred, and he didn't experience hunger or sugar cravings throughout the process.

Thyroid Hormones

Think of your thyroid as the "check engine" light on your vehicle. When it illuminates, you can keep driving for a few days without issues, sometimes even a few weeks if you push it. However, in the long term, it means something is off and you'll need to deal with it before it snowballs into a much bigger issue. Signs that may indicate it's time to get your thyroid checked include: a substantial increase in your weight (without any changes to your diet or exercise routine), feelings of extreme fatigue, missed periods, skin irritation or swelling, thinning hair, or even an overwhelming feeling of sadness or depression. If you are experiencing these symptoms, the best way to determine whether you have a thyroid issue is to screen for TSH (thyroid stimulating hormone) levels in your blood. In this case, high readings indicate low thyroid function. A healthy range for TSH is between 0.5 and 5.0 mIU/L, while a doctor will consider anything over 4.5 mIU/L to be a sign of an underactive thyroid. Anything 0.5 mIU/L or lower indicates an overactive thyroid.

Thyroid disease is serious and often requires medicine or medical intervention to treat, so be sure to consult with your doctor if you suspect you have thyroid issues.

Thyroid disease can also affect your carb tolerance, so here are the best strategies to take if you are diagnosed with overactive or underactive thyroid.

THE BEST CARBOHYDRATE APPROACH
FOR HYPOTHYROIDISM

When you have low thyroid production, your body is in an energy crisis. You feel so weak and tired, it's a struggle to sustain the energy for even basic functions, let alone working out. In this case, you cannot, I repeat, *cannot,* apply the same principles as someone with a healthy metabolism. In addition to low energy levels, common symptoms of low thyroid production are dry skin, feeling cold, low libido, heavy periods, brittle nails, constipation, and, last but not least, unexplained weight gain.

It's rare for a person to have a thyroid problem that stems from an issue with the thyroid gland itself. Over 90 percent of the time, thyroid issues stem from underlying health concerns. Because of this, there is a lot of debate among nutrition researchers regarding the appropriate level of carbs for those with thyroid dysfunction. To understand the proper range of carb intake, we need to take a deeper dive into thyroid hormones, how they function, what impacts their optimal function, what the research says about them, and how that relates to your specific situation.

The thyroid gland at the front of your neck is responsible for controlling your metabolism and creating the thyroid hormones, T3 and T4. If the body is not creating enough of the thyroid hormones, this condition is referred to as hypothyroidism. Some of the thyroid hormone's function takes place in the gut, muscle, heart, and nerves, but the majority occurs in the liver. It follows that if your liver is unhealthy, you may experience hypothyroidism. Several things can impede healthy liver function, such as constipation, gallbladder surgery or impaired gallbladder function, adrenal stress, or iodine deficiencies. High levels of estrogen or estrogen dominance can also cause low thyroid hormone production, as these hormones compete for the same receptors. Because so many parts of the body interact with the thyroid, understanding how it relates to carb tolerance can be tricky.

A client of mine once told me, "Hypothyroidism feels like you literally have no metabolism." As you can imagine, this is not only terrible for fat loss, but it's an awful state to live in. The ultimate goal with hypothyroidism is to get the body to a point where the thyroid is running again. I know those of you struggling with this issue are most concerned about weight gain, but before you can focus on losing weight, you need to get to a point where you feel better.

In fact, the *worst* thing you can do with hypothyroidism is go on a very low-calorie diet. When you eat below the level of calories your body needs to function, the body lowers your metabolism, and you burn fewer calories. The second worst thing you can do is consume the wrong types of calories. If you have hypothyroidism, you must eliminate inflammatory carbs, specifically gluten, dairy, and soy, and foods that inhibit iodine production, such as cruciferous vegetables and nitrates.[6] Outside of that, it's critical to have the correct approach to carbs.

In a long-term study called the Vermont Study, researchers found that changes in diet trigger corresponding changes in thyroid hormone levels.[7] Specifically, they found that increased caloric intake leads to increased levels of the T3 hormone. Their overall conclusion, which further studies have confirmed, is that carbohydrates are essential for optimal thyroid function.[8][9] For this reason, there is some cause for concern for people with hypothyroidism using very low-carb approaches.

T3 levels will drop if you are undereating, regardless of carb intake. However, specific carbs can introduce gut inflammation, which can further reduce thyroid hormone levels. This can make it seem as though you need to go low-carb, when in fact it's these inflammatory foods, not your carb levels, that are causing the problems.

There are different schools of thought when it comes to the right carbohydrate level for hypothyroidism. Some experts advocate for very low-carb, specifically keto, approaches because the thinking is that most low-calorie diets tend to be low-carb as well, and the lower T3 levels aren't such a bad thing if it leads to much desired weight loss.

That said, I don't recommend keto as the starting point if you have hypothyroidism. Very low-carb protocols are not always sustainable for the long haul, and just because you might be able to lose weight for a few months, it does not mean you will be able to keep it off. In addition, if gaining lean muscle is a goal of yours, you may experience challenges with workout recovery. I have had clients with hypothyroidism thrive on the ketogenic diet, but it's important to note that they paired this lifestyle with supervised medication from a doctor and had to adhere to it for years. In my experience, they are the exception and not the rule.

I suggest starting by eliminating refined carbs and inflammatory foods to return proper function to your thyroid. If your condition still does not improve after finding a careful balance of macros, I would suggest exploring a ketogenic approach, but only as a last resort. I am more concerned with your sustaining progress in the long term, not just losing a few quick pounds when your overall health may still be compromised.

THE BEST CARBOHYDRATE APPROACH
FOR HYPERTHYROIDISM

Unlike hypothyroidism, hyperthyroidism is when the thyroid produces excess thyroid hormone. The primary cause of hyperthyroidism is a condition known as Graves' disease, an autoimmune condition where antibodies overpromote hormone production. People have described hyperthyroidism as feeling like their "metabolism is on steroids." This condition is associated with weight loss, which you may think is a good thing, but if it goes untreated, it can lead to serious health concerns such as heart issues and fragile bones. Signs of hyperthyroidism include elevated heart rate, diarrhea, unexpected weight loss, and sweating. Many studies have established that hyperthyroidism is connected to insulin resistance.[10] Excess thyroid hormone can throw off glucose homeostasis, resulting in a change in the way your body processes carbs.

Nutritionally, the best thing you can do to address hyperthyroidism is consume targeted micronutrients such as foods that are low in iodine and high in calcium, selenium, iron, and vitamin D. Because carbs can raise thyroid hormone production, it makes sense that a customized ketogenic-style diet is effective for people with hyperthyroidism. However, if you don't feel comfortable committing to a ketogenic lifestyle, a low-carb nutrition plan that is free of caffeine, gluten, and cruciferous veggies will also work well. Limiting carb intake is the most practical approach to get this condition under control and promotes a lower carb tolerance.

Digestive Enzymes

One in four people experience indigestion on a regular basis.[11] Associated with symptoms such as an uncomfortable feeling of fullness after a meal, bloating, or even nausea with overeating, we tend to think indigestion isn't a serious condition. However, these symptoms can be early warning signs that there is an underlying issue.

Digestive enzymes are a crucial part of metabolizing carbohydrates. Amylase, the digestive enzyme that helps break down carbs into glucose, begins its work the moment carbs hit your tongue. If your mother ever told you to chew your food before swallowing, she may not have realized it, but she was helping you absorb carbs by giving your salivary amylase enzymes more time to work. As it only lasts a few seconds, we often overlook the practical importance of this predigestion stage, but it sets the stage for pancreatic amylase to finish the process of breaking carbs into glucose as they pass through the small intestine.

Amylase varies in amount from person to person. A low amylase level translates to a lower carb tolerance, and there is a higher carb tolerance when amylase levels are high. Research shows that low amylase levels are a major contributing factor to obesity, metabolic syndrome, and type 2 diabetes.[12] Digesting carbs is much more difficult for individuals with low amylase levels. On the flip side, digesting carbs is a breeze for those with adequate levels of this amylase.

Before you order a box of amylase enzymes online, remember that a high amylase level is not a free pass to eat carbs with abandon. Amylase supplements are ideal for relieving digestive discomfort in those with obvious carb tolerance issues or for occasional help digesting if you've consumed more than your body can handle.

The main determinant of amylase level is genetics, but there are cases where lifestyle factors such as alcoholism, eating disorders, and consistent low-quality nutrition can cause abnormal amylase levels. Still, for the majority of people, salivary and pancreatic amylase levels are genetic, meaning their ability to tolerate carbs may not owe to just diet and exercise alone. For those of you unable to lose weight even with regular exercise and clean eating, your genetic amylase level may be the reason why.

You can measure this predisposition with genetic testing. The main gene that determines your quantity of salivary amylase is known as AMY1. Individuals with more copies of the AMY1 gene produce more salivary amylase and have a higher carb tolerance as a result. Researchers have found a direct correlation between the number of AMY1 copies and how long ago a person's ancestors transitioned from hunter-gatherers to agriculture-based societies.[13] Agricultural societies such as Asian farming societies have evolved to have more copies of the AMY1 gene and thus higher carb tolerance levels. Conversely, those with low amylase levels have an inherited dietary history where their ancestors depended more on fatty acids as a fuel source.[14]

Gut Health

It's easy to confuse a gut health issue with a carb intolerance. For instance, you eat pancakes for breakfast, and before lunch you are already experiencing gas and bloating. This doesn't mean the only way for you to avoid this is to cut out carbs. The root cause of most gut health issues is a bacteria imbalance. When I see a client experiencing bloating, indigestion, a fat-loss plateau, or unexpected weight gain in a caloric deficit (when it's not that time of the month), I zero in on their reactions to specific foods before deciding to shift their macro ratios.

Complications in the gut arise as a result of inflammation. This may come as the result of drinking excess alcohol, taking antibiotics, smoking, getting insufficient sleep, feeling excess stress, or eating processed, refined foods. Over time, this can lead to leaky gut syndrome, where the gut lining begins to deteriorate, causing a high degree of permeability from the gut to the bloodstream. When this happens, harmful ingredients can leach into the bloodstream, resulting in inflammation. If you've got leaky gut, it is best to avoid whole grains, gluten, dairy, refined sugars, processed meats, and soy because they can be inflammatory. This does not always mean you should go low-carb, which can be easy to do by accident when you're eliminating these common carb sources.

Managing an autoimmune condition can be challenging and can make navigating weight loss even more challenging. Medication alone is not enough to manage an autoimmune disorder, and nutrition can be your greatest ally or biggest enemy.

Understanding food triggers is essential to reducing inflammation, and it's far more complicated than just staying away from foods that are obviously bad for you, like processed and refined foods. When the bacteria in your gut are off balance, the body can't regulate blood sugar and absorb nutrients at optimal capacity. When this happens, the main objective is to manage your overall gut bacteria by eliminating foods that introduce unfavorable bacteria and eating foods that reduce inflammation. This means eliminating dairy, soy, gluten, grains, and corn-fed meat, as well as nightshades and high-FODMAP foods. FODMAP is an acronym for fermentable oligio-, di-, mono-saccharides, and polyols — these are a very specific class of carbohydrate molecules that tend to disrupt healthy gut function.[15] If you experience common digestive issues like bloating, distended abdomen, IBS, painful gas, and even diarrhea, try shifting your diet toward low-FODMAP foods.[16] The average person looking at a list of high-FODMAP foods would be shocked to see items that seem clean and healthy — like garlic, onions, apples, mangos, cauliflower, and asparagus — are among an exhaustive list of foods that should be avoided, at least temporarily, until you get your gut back in balance. Be aware that for many people with issues such as these, there may be no going back to FODMAP foods without discomfort.

This is where working with a nutritionist can be very helpful in aiding you with cherry-picking the carbs that do not inflame your gut. While there may be anecdotal evidence showing that going very low-carb or even keto may be helpful for those with autoimmune diseases, it's not actually that simple. Going low-carb lowers insulin. Lowering insulin levels when the immune system is compromised can further complicate the endocrine system, which requires insulin for its vital roles. It is best to start with a moderate amount of noninflammatory carbs as a jumping-off point.

What's Your Carb Tolerance?

Each person has a tipping point where carb intake goes from a *good* thing that helps build muscle to outpacing the body's ability to metabolize it so that insulin becomes a fat-storing hormone. How much carb consumption leads to this point varies from person to person based on their overall carb tolerance, how much exercise they get, and how much energy their activity levels demand. If you are consuming more carbohydrates than you burn, and you aren't performing resistance training to a level that challenges your muscles to grow, your body will store these excess carbs as fat for future energy use.

So how much is too much? The amount of glycogen that the body can store will vary from person to person. One nice side effect of training is these limits actually go up when you add muscle mass! An average adult's total glycogen storage capacity is between 400 and 700 grams (which is between 1,600 and 2,800 calories of carbs). About 80 percent of those calories are stored in the muscle cells; the remainder is stored in the liver, with trace amounts stored in the blood. With intense training greater than 90 minutes per day, you can increase your glycogen storage capacity by about 15 percent.

If you don't work out regularly or if you *never* train to a level that requires your body to tap into your carbohydrate stores, any carb consumption above your personal glycogen threshold will be stored as fat. It's important to keep this perspective in mind when thinking about how many calories you need to burn to deplete your carb stores. Most people *overestimate* how many calories they burn from activity and *underestimate* how many carbs they are actually consuming. What you may think is low carb tolerance may actually be nothing more than unconsciously going over your carb limits and not being active enough. On the other hand, if you are actually being mindful about the quality and quantity of carbs consumed *and* you are exercising consistently *and* you are still experiencing challenges with fat loss, you may actually have a lower-than-average tolerance to carbohydrates.

Identifying an effective way to gauge whether or not you have a legitimate carb intolerance can be a challenge. Discovering your carb tolerance level is about recognizing the subtle nuances of your biological responses to certain foods. To help you establish where you fall on the spectrum of carb tolerance, I've provided this self-assessment quiz. It is an excellent starting point for uncovering the most appropriate way to nourish and fuel your body using science.

CARB TOLERANCE QUIZ

Answer the following questions, and keep track of the number of points assigned to each response.

1. What is your waist measurement at the smallest part of your waist (2 to 3 inches above the navel)?

    A. Under 30 inches (for females), under 35 inches (for males) [0 points]

    B. Under 35 inches (for females), under 40 inches (for males) [2 points]

    C. At 35 inches (for females), at 40 inches (for males) [3 points]

    D. Over 35 inches (for females), at 40 inches (for males) [5 points]

2. Where do you tend to gain weight?

    A. I gain weight evenly throughout my body. [0 points]

    B. I gain weight with more concentration in my hips, glutes, legs. [2 points]

    C. I gain weight with more concentration in my torso and have a "belly" when overweight. [5 points]

3. What is your waist-to-hip ratio? (Applies to women)
    WHR = waist measurement ÷ hip measurement
    (ex: 35-inch waist ÷ 42-inch hips = 0.83 WHR)

    A. Under 0.7 [0 points]

    B. 0.7 to 0.8 [0 points]

    C. 0.8 to 0.9 [1 point]

    D. 0.9 to 1.0 [3 points]

    E. Over 1.0 [5 points]

4. Have you ever been diagnosed with any of the following:

    A. Type 2 diabetes/prediabetes/insulin resistance [5 points]

    B. PCOS (polycystic ovarian syndrome) [4 points]

    C. Hypothyroidism [3 points]

    D. None of the above [0 points]

5. Do any of the following diseases run in your family?

    A. Obesity [1 point]

    B. High cholesterol [1 point]

    C. Type 2 diabetes [4 points]

    D. None of the above [0 points]

6. When you eat starchy carbs (i.e., rice, grains, potatoes, etc.), how long before you feel hungry again?

    A. I am full and satisfied until my next meal within 2 to 4 hours. [0 points]

    B. I am satisfied for about 60 minutes, but after that I could eat again. [2 points]

    C. I feel hungry again in about 30 minutes. [3 points]

    D. Once my hunger is turned "on," it never seems to be satisfied after I start, and I experience sugar cravings that continuously escalate. [5 points]

7. How does your digestive system respond after you eat starchy carbs?

    A. I do not have any issues digesting starchy carbs. [0 points]

    B. I experience occasional bloating but have normal digestion and bowel movements. [1 point]

    C. I experience bloating and digestive discomfort after consuming specific starchy carbs (i.e., gluten), but not all carbs. [3 points]

D. I experience bloating, gas, indigestion, inflammation, and irregular bowel movements after consuming *any* type of starchy carb or sugar. [4 points]

8. Have you been diagnosed with any of the following gut issues:

    A. SIBO (small intestinal bacterial overgrowth) [3 points]

    B. Leaky gut syndrome [3 points]

    C. IBS (irritable bowel syndrome) [3 points]

    D. None of the above [0 points]

    E. I'm not sure. I think I might, but I haven't been diagnosed. [2 points]

9. How do starchy carbs impact your cognitive energy?

    A. I can focus without any issues. [0 points]

    B. I lose focus easily but can push through if I consciously eliminate distractions. [1 point]

    C. I experience brain fog and am unable to work productively due to mental fatigue. [2 points]

    D. I feel the need to take a nap and can't function mentally without resting my mind first. [3 points]

10. How do carbs impact your physical energy?

    A. My energy is stable after I eat starchy carbs. [0 points]

    B. I feel tired when I overeat starchy carbs. [1 point]

    C. I feel like I need a nap within 1 to 2 hours of eating starchy carbs. [2 points]

11. Do you have a hard time controlling starchy carb and/or refined carb intake?

    A. I don't have any issues controlling my carb intake. [0 points]

B. Sometimes [2 points]

C. Yes, once I start, I cannot stop. [3 points]

12. What symptoms do you experience between meals?

A. I don't experience any symptoms; in fact, sometimes I forget to eat! [0 points]

B. I feel a little anxious but can deal if I drink water. [1 point]

C. I feel lightheaded, shaky, irritable, and/or anxious if I go without eating for longer than 4 hours. [2 points]

D. I feel lightheaded, shaky, irritable, and/or anxious if I go without eating longer than 2 hours. [4 points]

13. What best describes your sugar cravings?

A. I don't experience sugar cravings at all. [0 points]

B. I don't experience sugar cravings when I eat healthy balanced meals. [1 point]

C. I crave sweets during that time of the month, but other than that, not really. [2 points]

D. I crave sugar and sweets on a daily basis, regardless of if I just ate or not. [4 points]

14. Do you feel like you *must* eat before exercising?

A. No, I have no problem training in the fasted state, ever. [0 points]

B. Yes, but only if I'm weight training. [1 point]

C. Yes, I'll lose steam during my workout if I don't eat first. [2 points]

D. Yes, I'll get dizzy or nauseous if I don't eat before cardio and/or weight training. [2 points]

15. Do you feel you need to carry food/snacks with you because you are afraid you will get hungry?

    A. No, this has never even crossed my mind. [0 points]

    B. No, but this would help on long days. [1 point]

    C. Yes, I tend to need snacks throughout the day to balance energy and hunger. [2 points]

    D. Yes, if I don't, I will feel extremely hungry and will most likely overeat at the next meal. [3 points]

16. Do you eat a very clean diet with modest portions of healthy carbs and *still* are not able to lose weight?

    A. No, I can lose weight relatively easily simply by staying active. [0 points]

    B. No, but I can lose weight when I simply watch my portions regardless of what I eat. [1 point]

    C. Yes, even when my portions are dialed in, I still *struggle* to lose weight. [3 points]

    D. Yes, even with small portions of healthy carbs, I *cannot* lose weight. [5 points]

17. Do you experience any of these hormonal issues?
(Include all that apply to you.)

    A. Extremely heavy, irregular, or severely painful periods that last longer than 5 to 7 days [2 points]

    B. Hot flashes or night sweats [3 points]

    C. Mood swings, low libido, or severe PMS [2 points]

    D. Infertility [3 points]

    E. None of the above [0 points]

18. How would you describe the degree of difficulty you have when trying to lose weight?

    A. I have no issues at all; I'm naturally lean and tend to struggle to gain weight. [0 points]

    B. I gain weight easily, but I also lose it easily when I am focused. [1 point]

    C. I struggle to lose weight; I have to be extremely dedicated to see *any* progress. [2 points]

    D. I struggle to lose weight even when eating clean with 100 percent dedication and only seem to make *any* progress when I reduce my carb intake. [4 points]

19. Do you have intolerances to any of the following?

    A. Lactose [2 points]

    B. Gluten [2 points]

    C. Cruciferous veggies [1 point]

    D. Specific fruits [1 point]

    E. None of the above [0 points]

Now, add up the total points of all your answers. Use the key to see where you land.

Under 9 Points: High Carb Tolerance

You don't struggle to lose weight, and you can readily incorporate healthy carbs (and even refined carbs) without any issues. You may even be undereating carbs for your goal. When you consume carbs, you feel energized, satiated, and you do not experience any issues with blood sugar management. You thrive on carbs and are actually able to make even more progress on a moderate to moderately high ratio of carbs relative to the other macronutrient ratios.

UNLOCKING YOUR MACRO TYPE: REAL STORIES, REAL SUCCESSES

Sam, Carb-Fueled Macro Type

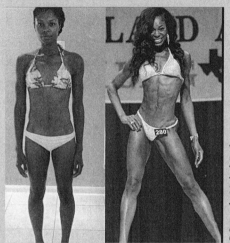

Before   *After*

When Sam and I started working together, she had a hard time adding lean muscle mass. Sam is an ectomorph with a naturally slender physique. Before we started working together, she was a distance runner and yoga enthusiast who ate between 1,000 and 1,200 calories per day. She was predominantly plant-based, so the majority of her calories came from carbs. We upped her daily caloric intake to 1,800 to 2,300 calories per day over the course of 12 weeks, which is approximately a 100 percent increase. This facilitated the growth of lean muscle mass while supporting body fat loss. She incorporated fish on this program to make it easier for her to hit the protein macros. She was not only pleased with her progress but shocked at how increased carbs allowed her to reach new levels of leanness while filling out her leg and glute muscles.

10 to 18 Points: Moderate Carb Tolerance

You can gain weight easily, but you can also lose it easily when you are focused and dialed in. You do need to pay attention to the quantity and type of carbs you consume, but you can include them in your diet without compromising your ability to lose body fat (therefore leading to a more sustainable lifestyle). On occasion, you struggle with cravings for sweets, but it's not a persistent situation. When you start eating more refined carbs, you do tend to crave them more and more, but when you dial it back and eat healthy carbs from real whole foods, you feel just fine. You only experience bloating and issues when you consume too many carbs or if you consume a specific carb that you have an intolerance to.

18 to 26 Points: Moderately Low Carb Tolerance

You gain weight easily and tend to struggle to drop weight even when you are focused and dialed in. You may be prediabetic, have hormonal issues, or have a slower overall metabolism. You have tried to cut out carbs to lose weight but can't sustain it, don't feel your best under those conditions, and experience low energy when you go too low in carbs. You have tried several diets and still can't pinpoint the correct approach to optimize your progress in a way that you can actually live with. If you have starchy carbs with every single meal, you know you will be bloated. As much as you enjoy carbs, you tend to experience better results when your carb intake is a little on the lower side.

Over 27 Points: Very Low Carb Tolerance

You feel like you have been struggling to lose weight for most of your life, or after a certain age or life event everything changed for you. When you consume moderate amounts of healthy carbs, you bloat, feel fatigued, and experience brain fog regularly. You experience persistent sugar cravings, you feel constantly hungry even if you just ate, and you struggle to satisfy your appetite with moderate amounts of food. You always feel like you could eat, and you snack so much that you may not even realize you are doing it. You experience digestive issues with particular carbs and feel immediately bloated when you consume them. At this point, you are open to trying anything that will help you, because everything you try doesn't seem to work.

Now that you have discovered, or perhaps confirmed, what your instincts told you about your carb tolerance, we are going to use this information to aid in defining your specific macro type. If you are on the cusp between two carb tolerance levels, I advise you to lean toward *higher* carbs as opposed to lower. It's best to test the upper limit of your carb tolerance so you can gauge how many carbs your body can handle. You can always reduce your carb intake if needed to facilitate progress. I don't advise going low-carb unless your body requires you to.

Keep in mind that your carb tolerance can change over time. This means that after a period of going very low to low-carb, your insulin resistance will improve, enabling you to tolerate a higher carb intake. This results in greater food freedom where you can incorporate carbs without weight gain. Carb tolerance levels can also regress. Just because you were once able to eat a very high carb intake without it impacting your body fat doesn't mean you will stay that way. Hormone imbalances, overconsumption of processed starches, and a sedentary way of life can lower carb tolerance as well.

I don't look at myself as a nutritionist; instead I see myself as the architect that you've hired to help you build the body of your dreams from the ground up. When someone decides to build a home, they tend to be primarily concerned with the aesthetics of the end project. Likewise, people tend to focus on outward appearance as a way to measure their success with a fitness program. You want an aesthetically pleasing figure, but as the biochemical architect of your body's remodel, I need to be sure that the home we are building can safely and sustainably function from the inside out. This is why we absolutely *need* to know these foundational internal factors about your carb tolerance. Imagine what a disaster it would be if an architect just plopped a premade design on your lot of land without surveying the land and assessing the type of soil, climate, etc. Unfortunately, this happens regularly with diet and fitness advice, which often is misaligned to the most important home you will ever own . . . your body! Let's make sure we take the utmost care of your body.

· · ·

Now that we know your carb tolerance, I am going to help you further define your macro type by figuring out which of the three macro nutrients — carbohydrates, protein, or fat — you need to consume the most and in what ratios. Armed with this information, you will be empowered to support your most functional health by dialing in the most appropriate macronutrient ratios to support your goals and help you get the best results while saving time and energy!

5

Identify Your Macro Type

Any plan detailed in any diet book that has ever been written worked well for the individual who wrote the book. But not every diet works for every person due to our unique biological profiles. In order to obtain and sustain results, you've got to pick the plan that will be the best fit for *you*.

Think of each nutrition plan as the blueprint to build a specific type of home. Imagine you picked up the plans to build a beautiful Tahitian hut. Only you don't live in Tahiti; you live in the mountains of Alaska. An open-air, bamboo hut with a thatched roof would be glorious in a hot climate. But that same structure located in an environment with ice, snow, and subzero temperatures: not so nice. You wouldn't make it through the first night. Yet this is what we do all the time when we try to adopt nutrition protocols that are not designed to handle the environmental factors of your specific body. Your nutritional home needs to be constructed of materials that fit the environment of your body, not someone else's.

If you have ever struggled to see results after following a nutrition plan that did wonders for a friend, you probably assumed that you did something wrong. You might have come away feeling terribly discouraged and thinking that you would never be able to drop the weight no matter what, so you might as well just say "f*** it." You can set those feelings down. You didn't fail because you lacked willpower or you didn't try hard enough. The diet failed you because it was not designed for *your* unique physiology and biochemical needs. In other words, it wasn't a match for your macro type. In this chapter, I'm going to help you figure out your macro type so you never have to go through that again.

When I started working with Hannah, she was one bad diet away from throwing in the towel and opting for liposuction and a tummy tuck. Hannah was a working mom in her 30s, and she hadn't felt confident in her body since before she had kids. She had never been thin and was naturally curvy and voluptuous her entire adult life. While Hannah loved her curves, she felt uncomfortable in a bathing suit because of her tummy. She was so self-conscious about her upper arms, she always wore long sleeves, especially when someone was going to take her picture.

She'd had some success on a "bro diet" that a bodybuilder had created for her before she had her youngest child. This diet consisted of preportioned containers of dry chicken breast, broccoli, and modest portions of sweet potatoes. While it got results, it was not only unsustainable, but it was also boring, bland, and joyless. Every health guru she met with told her to "eat this and not that," but they didn't help her dial in her caloric intake, nor did they look at her macros. Hannah knew she was eating healthy, clean, organic foods, but weight loss still eluded her.

By the time she reached out to me, she was beyond frustrated. When I screened her, we established that she has a moderately low carb tolerance (even though she loves carbs), but it wasn't so low that she needed to be on a keto diet. We determined that she would do better with a slightly higher-fat approach. Last but not least, we discovered that she only needs a moderate amount of protein, so the bro diet was a no-go for her health goals. The plan we created for her was completely differ-ent from the extreme diets she was familiar with, like high-protein/low-fat approaches and high-fat/low-carb diets such as keto.

Hannah's story turned out to be an *epic* success. The first three to four days were challenging for her as she got used to her appropriate portions. But eating for her macro type enabled her to break a five-year plateau in her weight, and she dropped 14 pounds in twelve weeks. She kept her normal day-to-day routine, which included low to moderate activity and light exercise. The big shift was sticking to her customized nutrition plan, which included things like salmon, avocado toast, pro-tein pancakes, occasional pasta and pizza, chicken wings, salads, veg-gies, rice, and even cream in her coffee every day! Hannah was blown away by all the foods she *could* eat while still making progress toward her goals. She told me that for the first time, she didn't feel like she was on a diet. She never imagined that she could eat foods she enjoyed while getting results.

Sound exciting?

Let's back up a bit so I can explain how macro typing allowed Han-nah to experience such great results. Then I'll help you pinpoint your macro type so you can get started on the best eating plan for you.

All About Macros

As a refresher, macronutrients, aka macros, are the nutrients that the body requires in large quantities: protein, carbohydrates, and fat. Every diet, at its core, is a nutritional guide containing varying ratios of pro-teins, carbs, and fats. For instance, a traditional vegan diet eliminates meat, seafood, poultry, dairy, and eggs. While a vegan diet doesn't dic-tate specific macronutrient ranges, it tends to be higher in carbs, lower in fat, and very low in protein. Or take the paleo diet. Since this eating style eliminates gluten, grains, dairy, processed sugars, legumes, and soy, it tends to be lower in carbs and higher in healthy fats even though there are no assigned macronutrient ranges that require this to be the case.

No diet is inherently bad, and certainly opting to eat more whole foods over processed foods is a great thing. But you will struggle to get results on any diet plan if it's not the right diet for *you*. This is why you need to match your eating plan to your macro type. In this chapter, I'm going to help you discover the balance of macronutrients *your* body needs. When you know your target percentage of protein, carbs, and fat, you can align what you eat with what your body needs.

Once you identify your macro type, you can optimize your nutrient intake to meet your health goals. Most of my clients are surprised to find they get to eat more of certain nutrients than they thought was possible. Don't get hung up on what you can't have; instead focus on what you can have. You may be able to eat more carbs than you realized; you may need to eat far fewer carbs but get to consume much more fat. The important thing to remember is that you're getting a key that will unlock your body's best response to food and help you lose fat in a healthy and lasting way.

Don't spend another minute fighting your body with a plan that doesn't work for you. Once you eat for your macro type, I guarantee you can achieve your health goals, and you'll feel an improved sense of self-care.

WHY THE USDA IS GIVING YOU BAD ADVICE

Before we go any further, let's first acknowledge the fact that the USDA's dietary recommendations apply to only about 20 percent of women and 30 to 35 percent of men. In other words, the USDA's Recommended Daily Allowances (RDAs) are contrary to what roughly 70 to 80 percent of Americans need. This comes as a shock to most people.

The disconnect stems from the fact that the USDA's recommended carb-dominant approach is only suitable for active individuals seeking to maintain an already healthy weight.

Take a look around on your next trip to your local grocery store, and you will see clear evidence that the average American is far above a healthy weight. The USDA standards are not based on an accurate representation of what the average American needs to regain their health.

The ability to lose body fat without losing lean muscle mass is all about eating an appropriate amount of protein to sustain a positive nitrogen balance. The body requires this condition to burn fat for fuel when in a caloric deficit. However, determining just how much protein you need can be a confusing subject, as there are many different standards for determining dietary protein intake.

According to the USDA, the daily recommended value for protein based on a diet of 2,000 calories per day is 50 grams, or 10 percent of your total calories. The problem with this standard is that the USDA bases this calculation on the nitrogen balance the body needs to maintain its basic functions and support DNA synthesis. The USDA has no guidelines explaining how much quality protein a person requires to support basic activity, resistance training, stress, blood sugar support, or to help stabilize muscle and blood sugar with age. It doesn't account for the protein a person loses due to training, the role of protein as a signaling molecule to maintain an efficient metabolism, or the amount of protein a person needs to maintain lean muscle mass.

The rule of thumb in the bodybuilding community is to consume

1 gram of protein per pound of lean body mass per day, which is a reasonable ballpark value to support muscle growth. In-depth nitrogen balance studies have shown that athletes and bodybuilders need 1.7 g/kg of protein per pound of body weight.[1] Other studies have shown elite powerlifters can gain strength when they boost their daily dietary protein intake from 1.7 to 3.5 g/kg per pound of body weight over the course of several months of weight training. Now, not everyone is trying to break a world weightlifting record, but everyone can benefit from a protein intake of 1 gram of protein per pound of your target body weight to support a positive nitrogen balance. The USDA's recommendation of only 50 grams of protein per day, or 10 percent of your total daily caloric intake, is *much* lower than what any nutritionist with practical experience would advise.

So, What's Your Macro Type?

Now for the fun part—time to identify your macro type. There are five distinct macro types, differentiated into three primary categories— Carb-Fueled, Protein-Fueled, and Fat-Fueled. There are two subcategories for the protein- and fat-fueled types based on carb tolerance (Protein-Fueled/Low-Carb and Fat-Fueled/Low-Carb). While the protein- and fat-fueled types will never require a high-carb diet, some people will thrive with a moderate-carb intake, while others will need to restrict their carb intake to lower levels in order to see results and feel their best.

This quiz consists of carefully designed questions to help you assess your specific macro type. Read each question carefully, and score yourself based on the response that best describes your *current situation*—not your ideal situation, not how you used to be, not how you feel "sometimes" — but the reality of your current circumstances. Your macro type is based on your total score at the end of the quiz. If your score is on the borderline between two macro types, read the descriptions of each type, and go with the one that you believe best fits your current circumstances.

Once you've taken the quiz and found your macro type, I'll describe each of the five types in detail. By the end of this chapter, you should have a pretty good sense of your type and your personal best macro ratios.

FIND YOUR MACRO TYPE QUIZ

Answer the following questions and keep track of the number of points assigned to each response.

1. Based on your results from the Carb Tolerance Quiz in Chapter 4, what is your carb tolerance?

     A. High carb tolerance (0 points)

     B. Moderate carb tolerance (3 points)

     C. Moderately low carb tolerance (6 points)

     D. Very low carb tolerance (12 points)

2. Has your gallbladder been removed?

     A. Yes, my gallbladder was removed, and I am *unable* to digest high-fat foods. (0 points)

     B. No, but I have gallstones and/or occasional pain when digesting high-fat foods. (3 points)

     C. Yes, my gallbladder was removed, but I am *able* to digest high-fat foods with meds and supplementation. (6 points)

     D. No, I have my gallbladder and have zero issues digesting fat. (6 points)

3. How easy is it for you to add lean muscle?

A. I struggle to add curves and shape to my frame. (0 points)

B. I can add lean muscle with intentional effort and have visible muscle definition when I am focused. (3 points)

C. I can add muscle pretty easily, but it's getting a little harder with age. (6 points)

D. I add muscle easily but wasn't thicker until adulthood or after kids. (9 points)

E. I bulk up quickly and have always been naturally on the thicker side. (12 points)

4. If the rate at which you dropped body fat was a mode of transportation, what would best describe it?

A. Private jet: It is never ever an issue to get to my destination with zero holdups. (0 points)

B. Commercial airline, nonstop: I have to deal with the hassle of security and getting to the airport early, but no issues to get to the destination once I'm aboard the plane. (3 points)

C. Commercial airline, multiple stops: I experience layovers here and there, and it typically takes me a little longer, but I always get there even if it means a little more hassle. (6 points)

D. Cancelled flight, need to rent a car: I'd fly if I could, but it's just not an option, so I need to rent a car. I'll get there some way somehow, even if it feels like it's going to be a while, and this is far from ideal. (9 points)

E. In a car, with a flat tire, on the side of the road . . . I'm okay driving as long as I can get there, but I'm beginning to wonder if I ever will. I can't even make progress until I get this flat fixed. (12 points)

5. What describes the vibe you get from others toward your health goals?

    A. *"Will you please eat a burger?! You need to eat!"* (0 points)

    B. *"You are already healthy; you don't need to be this obsessed."* (3 points)

    C. *"You aren't getting any younger, probably want to stay on top of that."* (6 points)

    D. *"Maybe you need to work out more."* (9 points)

    E. *"Maybe you should see a doctor."* (12 points)

6. What best describes your appetite?

    A. I struggle to eat and tend to get full easily. I even forget to eat at times. (0 points)

    B. I have a healthy appetite with occasional cravings but nothing major. (3 points)

    C. If I don't drink water and track my food intake, I can easily go over my daily calories without even realizing it. (6 points)

    D. I have a hard time keeping my appetite in check. (9 points)

    E. I crave carbs and sugar most of the time, and once I start eating carbs, I feel like I can't turn off my appetite. (12 points)

7. Can you lose weight while including starchy carbohydrates (bread, pasta, white potatoes) in your diet?

    A. Yes, I can eat "whatever" and never gain a pound. (0 points)

    B. Yes, as long as I'm working out regularly. (3 points)

    C. Yes, but it depends on the portions and frequency; I need to be mindful. (6 points)

    D. Not really. I can eat starches, but I can't have them every day. (9 points)

    E. I wish. I typically need to go very low in carbs to see any changes. (12 points)

8. Have you ever experienced any issues with an underactive thyroid (hypothyroidism)?

    A. No, but I do have hyperthyroidism/overactive thyroid. (0 points)

    B. Never. (0 points)

    C. Yes, but I'm on medication for it and am managing it without issues. (6 points)

    D. Yes, and I'm struggling with weight loss as a result of it. (9 points)

    E. No, but I have a sluggish metabolism. (12 points)

9. Which best describes your *current* build?

    A. Naturally slender and lean; when I stop working out, I tend to lose weight without trying. (0 points)

    B. Naturally muscular; when I stop working out and eating right, I tend to gain weight easily. (3 points)

    C. Moderate build; I need to stay active to maintain a healthy physique. (6 points)

    D. Naturally curvy or apple shaped; if I don't remain active, I will gain weight very easily. (9 points)

    E. Naturally thicker; I struggle to lose weight even when I am eating right and working out. (12 points)

10. Which best describes your physique as an adult (before kids or lifestyle-related weight gain)?

    A. Always been naturally thin and lean (0 points)

    B. Naturally athletic (3 points)

    C. Yo-yo, have never been able to sustain a healthy body for more than a few months at a time (6 points)

    D. Naturally curvy (9 points)

    E. Naturally thicker, have been overweight my entire adult life (12 points)

11. Have you ever been diagnosed with a kidney disorder?

    A. No, I've never experienced any issues with my kidneys. (0 points)

    B. No, but I've experienced kidney stones or gout. (6 points)

    C. Yes, my doctor specifically advised me to *avoid* high-protein diets. (9 points)

12. What type of breakfast would give you the most stable energy?

    A. Protein pancakes topped with sliced bananas and maple syrup (0 points)

    B. Egg whites, breakfast meat of choice, and a side of toast or small bowl of oats (3 points)

    C. Whole eggs, breakfast meat of choice, and a side of low-sugar fruit (6 points)

    D. Whole eggs, avocado, and mixed greens (12 points)

13. What type of snacks make you feel the best?

    A. Fresh fruit, granola (0 points)

    B. Protein smoothie with fresh fruit (3 points)

    C. Protein shakes, beef jerky, turkey breast (6 points)

    D. Hard-boiled eggs, nuts, seeds, etc. (9 points)

    E. Nuts, cheese, avocado (12 points)

14. What best describes your health goals?

    A. Maintain my body weight, gain lean muscle, and lose some fat (0 points)

    B. Lose 5 to 20 pounds and appear more defined, toned, and lean (3 points)

    C. Lose over 25 pounds of fat to start feeling healthy again (6 points)

    D. Lose fat, but mostly feel better again from a hormonal health perspective (9 points)

    E. Lose more than 50 pounds of stubborn fat (12 points)

15. Have you ever been diagnosed with a hormone imbalance?

    A. No, I have no issues, and my cycle is never ever late. (0 points)

    B. No confirmed imbalances, but I've experienced occasional irregular cycles that are shorter or longer in nature. (3 points)

    C. No imbalances, but I've lost my period before at times. (6 points)

    D. Yes, I've experienced estrogen dominance, PCOS, perimenopause, or menopause. (9 points)

    E. Yes, I'm struggling with type 2 diabetes. (12 points)

Now, add up the total points of all your answers. Use the key to see where you land.

Under 10 Points: Carb-Fueled Macro Type

10 to 40 Points: Protein-Fueled Macro Type

40 to 70 Points: Protein-Fueled/Low-Carb Macro Type

70 to 90 Points: Fat-Fueled Macro Type

90 to 150 Points: Fat-Fueled/Low-Carb Macro Type

Understanding Your Macro Type

Now that you've completed the quiz and got your score, I'm going to help you understand your macro type and give an explanation of each one. There are a total of five macro types, which comprise the most common recommended eating styles based on the relative ratios of the most dominant to the least dominant macronutrients. This simple system allows you to intuitively navigate the fundamental differences in each macro-based approach to nutrition. Once you know your macro type, you can easily see at a glance which range best supports your needs.

As you can see in the chart below, there are drastic differences in the relative ratios of proteins, carbs, and fats between the five macro types. This is why it's vital to align your eating style with your body's needs. (I've also provided the USDA's recommended daily allowance [RDA] ratios for comparison.)

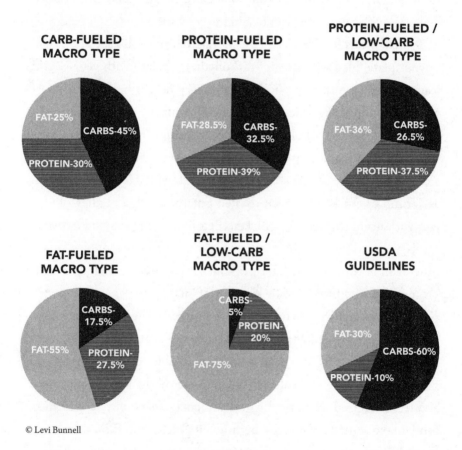

CARB-FUELED MACRO TYPE
FAT-25%
CARBS-45%
PROTEIN-30%

PROTEIN-FUELED MACRO TYPE
FAT-28.5%
CARBS-32.5%
PROTEIN-39%

PROTEIN-FUELED / LOW-CARB MACRO TYPE
FAT-36%
CARBS-26.5%
PROTEIN-37.5%

FAT-FUELED MACRO TYPE
CARBS-17.5%
FAT-55%
PROTEIN-27.5%

FAT-FUELED / LOW-CARB MACRO TYPE
CARBS 5%
PROTEIN-20%
FAT-75%

USDA GUIDELINES
FAT-30%
CARBS-60%
PROTEIN-10%

© Levi Bunnell

Now, here's the deep dive into each macro type, so you can begin to craft the perfect nutrition plan for yourself.

TYPE 1: CARB-FUELED MACRO TYPE

If your score was under 10 points or if you answered mostly A's, you are most aligned with the Carb-Fueled Macro Type. An ideal eating plan for this macro type consists of 45 percent carbs, 30 percent protein, and 25 percent fat. Of the three macronutrients, you do best when you consume a higher proportion of your total daily caloric intake from carbohydrates, with moderate protein and lower fat intake.

Typical meals for the Carb-Fueled Macro Type will have about half of your plate filled with quality carbohydrates paired with veggies and lean proteins, while going lighter on dietary fats. A healthy breakfast would include things like protein powder mixed into oatmeal, egg white omelets with whole grain toast and fruit, or protein pancakes topped with fruit. A healthy lunch or dinner would include things like a chicken-and-rice veggie stir-fry, a pasta dish with a lean protein such as shrimp or chicken, or oven-roasted potatoes with a medley of veggies with lean fish, steak, or chicken. Before working out and between meals, you will function best when snacking on bananas, apples, or another fruit of your choice. After workouts, it's optimal to include a high-protein shake with fruit, while keeping fat intake low.

If you have confirmed you are a Carb-Fueled Macro Type, this means you struggle to gain quality weight and have been naturally lean for most of your life. Quality foods with more carbs enable you to add curves to your frame for a fuller, healthier, and stronger body. You function best and feel energized when the highest percentage of your macronutrient food intake consists of healthy, high-quality carbs. You should embrace foods like whole grains, root vegetables, rice, potatoes, fruit, and vegetables. In most cases, this means you will be moderate with your protein intake and eat foods lower in dietary fats, which translates into leaner protein sources like whey isolate, chicken breast, white fish, shrimp, lean turkey, lean steak, egg whites, etc.

Many of the Carb-Fueled Macro Types I work with feel like they have struggled with their physique but not in the typical way. If you are carb-fueled, it may be that you have been picked on for years for being too thin or scrawny. People may mock you for wanting to improve your body composition, because to them you are already a "skinny mini." You know you are thin, but you have visible body fat (aka *skinny fat*) or you may be "softer" than you prefer and want to add muscle tone and definition, maybe even some feminine curves.

Carb-Fueled Macro Types tend to have a "fast" metabolism compared to the average person and have difficulty gaining weight regardless of how much they eat. They often are picky eaters with small appetites and in most cases have been thin their entire lives. This body type has a tiny bone structure, narrow shoulders, flat chest, narrow waist and hips, small wrists, skinny ankles, and an overall straight-lined body type. Sometimes, but not always, they're a bit on the lanky side, with longer-than-average limbs and longer-than-average bellies.

Every macro type can gain weight, but when a Carb-Fueled Macro Type gains weight, it tends to be "skinny-fat" weight gain, which translates to a high percentage of body fat and low muscle mass. Even at a healthy weight, they can still have a disproportionate amount of body fat, in most cases concentrated in the torso. This makes these macro types feel the need to work out harder and eat even less. But that's not the solution.

If this is you, your body loses fat with the most ease, and it requires less effort to transform its composition. Your biggest challenge will be eating more food. Yes, you read that correctly! What you need to do to get the lean, shapely physique you want may run counter to what you've been told. You need to be on a carb-dominant nutrition approach with dialed-in protein and fats to support your physical goals. Getting more of your calories from carbs will support you in gaining muscle by improving your recovery and fueling optimal physical performance. For the Carb-Fueled Macro Type, carbs provide the primary fuel source to train at maximum capacity, recover the most efficiently, and support muscle growth.

UNLOCKING YOUR MACRO TYPE: REAL STORIES, REAL SUCCESSES

Liz, Carb-Fueled Macro Type

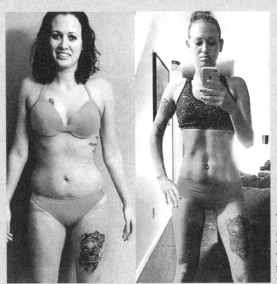

Before   *After*

© Elizabeth Josephs

Meet Liz, an ectomorph and bikini competitor. When she first took an interest in fitness competitions, she was already at a lean weight of 127 pounds at 5 foot, 7 inches, and a mother of two beautiful girls. The problem wasn't a need to lose weight, but she wanted to shift her body composition by dropping fat and adding muscle by increasing her calories and carb count significantly. She weighs the same in her before and after photos, but was able to drop her waist from 28 inches to 24 inches while gaining lean muscle and eating over 3,000 calories a day. Her body responded wonderfully to the shift in increased calories, increased carb content, and overall nourishment. This is a perfect example of how eating more carbs and more calories overall actually helped her drop body fat.

UNLOCKING YOUR MACRO TYPE: REAL STORIES, REAL SUCCESSES

Julie, Carb-Fueled Macro Type

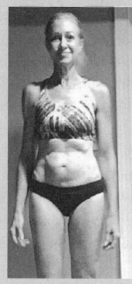 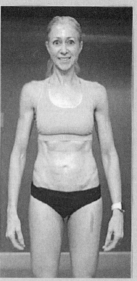

Before   *After*

Julie is a distance runner with a naturally slender physique. To most people, she is already tiny, and the idea of needing to optimize her nutrition may seem odd to most. However, she wanted to move away from a skinny fat physique to a strong, lean, and athletic figure. Julie wanted to reduce body fat and gain lean muscle. Her carb intake increased from only 130 grams to over 270 grams per day. She never would have done this on her own, as the concept of eating more carbs seemed unimaginable. She dropped 3.5 percent body fat in twelve weeks and went from a 26-inch waist to a 24-inch waist. She is a perfect example that more cardio and eating less does not equal fat loss. At 49 years young, she then was able to hit new PR's with her race times, and she has sustained her fat loss.

The carb-fueled eating plan is also excellent for elite athletes who require more fuel to sustain their training needs. But before you start loading up on carbs, let me define an elite athlete. High-level athletes tend to train a minimum of 2 hours a day, six days a week, and burn at least 1,000 calories a day from workouts alone. This is not to say you aren't doing a great job if you do less than 45 minutes of cardio or your weight training takes less than an hour; it just means you don't automatically fall under the carb-dominant macro type. Even some highly active people don't have the ability to optimize and thrive with a carb-dominant eating plan. However, most individuals with high levels of activity *do* fit these criteria. If you are performing more than 90 minutes of cardiovascular exercise daily, you most likely need a carb-dominant nutrition plan to compensate for the volume of calories you burn. This may also apply if you have a physically demanding job, such as a nurse who logs 15,000 to 20,000 steps per day, a construction worker, or a server who is on their feet for more than 8 hours a day.

Last but not least, the carb-dominant macro type eating plan is ideal if you are dying to add curves to your frame. You don't care about the scale; you want a *fit-thick* aesthetic. For women, this means you have no desire to look überthin and want fuller glutes and legs while maintaining a slimmer torso. Men want a fuller chest, back, and arms with a V shape from shoulders to waist. Your priority is to change your shape, and you want to have curves for days.

You may have attempted getting thicker in the past, but your efforts only resulted in a bloated midsection, and the parts of your body that you wanted to get bigger refused to grow. You may have given up and told yourself that the only way for you to improve your look is to just get lean, as the fit-thick thing will just not work for you. You know you need to eat healthy; you know you need to eat more; but what that translates to in real food perplexes you. If this is you, and you do not have a low carb tolerance related to diabetes, PCOS, insulin resistance, or a hormone imbalance, you will do best on a Carb-Fueled Macro Type plan.

TYPE 2: PROTEIN-FUELED MACRO TYPE

The protein-fueled way of eating is typically associated with methods common to fitness competitors and bodybuilders. An ideal eating plan for this macro type consists of 39 percent protein, 32.5 percent carbs, and 28.5 percent fat. Of the three macronutrients, you do best when you consume a higher proportion of your total daily caloric intake from protein, with moderate carbs and lower fat intake.

Typical meals for the Protein-Fueled Macro Type will have about half of your plate filled with quality proteins, paired with a moderate amount of veggies and starchy carbs, while keeping the fats light. A healthy breakfast would include things like an English muffin sandwich with turkey bacon and egg, protein and low-sugar fruit smoothies, or protein oatmeal. A healthy lunch or dinner would include something along the lines of a high-protein veggie stir-fry bowl, ground meat with sweet potatoes and veggies, or chicken fajitas. Before working out and between meals, you function best when snacking on high-protein snacks such as protein shakes, Greek yogurt, bone broth, beef jerky, cottage cheese, or string cheese. After workouts, it's optimal to include a high-protein shake with fruit, while keeping the fat intake low.

This is the approach many celebrities follow, from Instagram fitness models to people like J. Lo and The Rock. If you fit the Protein-Fueled Macro Type, you function best when a larger portion of your calories comes from protein. Why is protein such a game-changer for you? Protein is the only macronutrient that contains nitrogen. Shifting the body toward a positive nitrogen balance supports greater fat loss when in a caloric deficit.[2]

This plan is excellent for those with a healthy metabolism, moderate carb tolerance, and normal hormonal function who are looking to obtain a toned physique while reducing body fat. For those seeking a physique that is more muscular without being bulky, for women who want a fit yet feminine look, and for those who aspire toward the body of a fitness model (leaning toward visible abs), the protein-dominant approach is for you. About 40 to 50 percent of people with the Protein-Fueled Macro Type don't need to worry about what they eat with painstaking detail, as they can gain muscle mass and lose weight with relative ease. The biggest challenge of this eating style tends to be getting enough protein from lean sources. If you are used to eating whole eggs, this doesn't mean you have to cut them out; it means you need to pay attention to their fat content. Fats add up quickly in certain types of protein. You should limit foods like red meat, fatty fish, and nuts to modest portion sizes, and make foods like egg whites, lean chicken, fish, turkey, and protein supplements the major staples in your day.

This combination gives the Protein-Fueled Macro Type the capacity to achieve fantastic definition. The challenge for this macro type is they can gain weight just as easily as they can lose it. While this may not seem like an insurmountable problem, it can sneak up on you if you get complacent. This macro type tends to store fat relatively evenly, which is why fat gain tends to creep up unnoticed for a while, because this type doesn't tend to have a belly, even when slightly overweight. There are genetic exceptions, however.

UNLOCKING YOUR MACRO TYPE:
REAL STORIES, REAL SUCCESSES
Yasmin, Protein-Fueled Macro Type

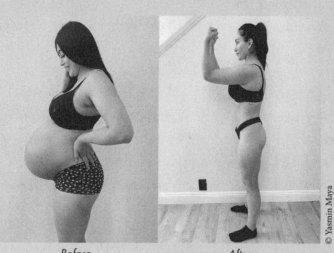

Before   *After*

© Yasmin Maya

I've had the privilege of supporting Yasmin through several stages of her health journey. She is a classic mesomorph who gains weight easily but also loses it easily. We started focusing on fat loss by dialing in her nutrition while making sure she didn't lose her curves. We then moved into lean gains, as she wanted to drop fat and add muscle while trying to conceive. Once she conceived, we had her on a healthy pregnancy plan and then supported her to postpregnancy, where she lost the baby weight and is thriving on her high-protein, low-fat, moderate-carb approach to nutrition. Her meal plans were simple, no-fuss, convenience-based meals. We found that her body does best when we dial up the protein and don't overdo it on the fats. Surprisingly enough, she does great with carbs and is able to add nice muscle tone when we make sure she keeps carbs in her diet.

. When you think of the Protein-Fueled Macro Type, think *lean muscle mass*. This is by far the most effective approach if your goal is to get super lean. If you are a woman plateaued between 15 and 23 percent body fat or a man plateaued between 10 and 18 percent and are looking to have visible abs (which entails getting down to 13 percent body fat for a woman and less than 10 percent for a man), this approach is ideal.

TYPE 3: PROTEIN-FUELED/LOW-CARB MACRO TYPE

This approach is ideal for those who struggle to stick to the traditional fitness competitor/bodybuilder nutrition plan due to the low fat content. An ideal eating plan for this macro type consists of 37.5 percent protein, 36 percent fat, and 26.5 percent carbs. Of the three macronutrients, you do best when you consume a higher proportion of your total daily caloric intake from protein, with moderate fat and lower carb intake.

Typical meals for the Protein-Fueled/Low-Carb Macro Type will have about 40 percent of your plate filled with fatty protein sources paired with lower GI carbs like cruciferous veggies, squash, or leafy greens cooked in a healthy fat source like olive oil. (GI stands for *glycemic index*. For more on the GI scale, see page 150.) A healthy breakfast would include things like salmon avocado toast, quiche, or whole eggs with leafy greens and a side of low-sugar fruit. A healthy lunch or dinner would include things like a rice bowl with veggies and a protein, salmon or chicken thighs with roasted squash and veggies, or oven-roasted potatoes with a medley of veggies with steak, chicken, or fatty fish. Before working out and between meals, you function best when snacking on bananas, apples, or any fruit of your choice. After workouts, it's optimal to include a high-protein shake with fruit while keeping the fat intake low.

If you fall into this category, you may not yet be at the point where you need medication to support hormone imbalances with respect to estrogen, progesterone, insulin, or thyroid issues, but you are beginning to notice inflammation, fatigue, or brain fog when you consume higher levels of carbs. Some clues that you may have a lower carb tolerance include the following: You'll notice you feel more satiated eating whole eggs as opposed to egg whites, chicken thighs as opposed to chicken breast, and you feel the need to have slightly higher levels of healthy fats in your meals to keep your appetite under control. This macro type tends to store their body fat evenly or in the lower half.

As a Protein-Fueled/Low-Carb Macro Type, you may suspect your metabolism is beginning to slow down with age or hormone shifts. This does not mean your metabolism is shot by any means, but you observe a higher sensitivity to inflammatory foods like gluten, grains, dairy, soy, and perhaps even select veggies. You may have been diagnosed with an autoimmune disease, and you may have days when you feel an overall sense of sluggishness that can't be cured with a cup of coffee. A protein-fueled/low-carb plan is also ideal for those who are beginning to experience irregular periods with respect to duration and cycle length but not necessarily missing periods. This is ideal for those who want the aesthetic of lean muscle mass and are looking to hit a goal of at least 20 to 23 percent body fat for women or 13 to 18 percent body fat for men.

UNLOCKING YOUR MACRO TYPE:
REAL STORIES, REAL SUCCESSES

Lory, Protein-Fueled/Low-Carb Macro Type

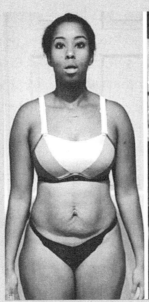 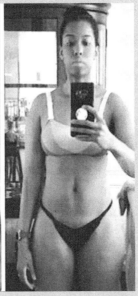

Before   After

Lory is a working mom of two who's been doing this program for a year and a half. While she doesn't have diabetes or insulin resistance, she has specific intolerances and sensitivities to lactose and high-FODMAP foods, which means she's better off eating a moderately low-carb plan (75 to 100 grams of carbs). She responded best with high protein, slightly lower carbs, and moderate to moderately low fat. When she started, her waistline was over 35 inches, and it's now under 26 inches — she's down almost 10 inches in her torso yet has maintained her curves. Every time people see these photos, they assume she had a tummy tuck; however, these incredible results are 100 percent from nutrition and consistent exercise.

When I think of the best nutrition plan for the Protein-Fueled/ Low-Carb Macro Type, I think of meals with fatty protein sources (like salmon, eggs, or chicken thighs), lots of veggies, and smaller portions of starchy carbs (2 to 3 ounces or less per meal). While you can consume these fatty proteins for any macro type, they tend to be a staple that this type is drawn to for its increased satiety effect. Many people who need a low-carb approach to lose weight often try the most extreme, restrictive version and give up. Even if you have a lower carb tolerance, you still *need* carbs. This eating style is about curating the correct foods to navigate your macros according to goals while relearning how to assemble fulfilling and satisfying meals. You may be relieved to learn that you can still consume carbs in moderation, but keep in mind that you can't afford to take extended breaks where you eat anything you want, as it will get harder and harder to keep your body fat down with age.

If you're this category, your margin of error is much smaller than the other macro types. If you don't keep your macros dialed in, you will experience prolonged plateaus. If you have a healthy but slightly declining metabolism and are starting to experience carb tolerance issues, this is by far the most effective approach to lean out. If you are a woman and your fat loss has plateaued between 25 and 32 percent body fat or are a man plateaued between 18 and 23 percent and are looking to get to the point where you can transition out of fat-loss mode and maintain a healthy body fat level under 25 percent for women and under 18 percent for men, this is the macro type plan you should follow.

TYPE 4: FAT-FUELED MACRO TYPE

I have found this to be the most neglected macro type, teeming with individuals who have been left feeling *stuck* when it comes to their health. I first noticed this macro type in clients over the age of 35 who did not respond well to the protein-fueled (aka high-protein/low-fat) approach that had worked so well for me. In 2015, I began to see more clients whose first priority was to feel better overall, followed shortly after by a desire to lose fat. (Many were coming off of quick-fix, results-oriented nutrition protocols that left them feeling hormonally or metabolically "off.") An ideal eating plan for this macro type consists of 55 percent fat, 27.5 percent protein, and 17.5 percent carbs. Of the three macronutrients, you do best when you consume a higher proportion of your total daily caloric intake from fat, with moderate protein and lower carb intake.

Typical meals for the Fat-Fueled Macro Type will have over half of your plate filled with fatty protein sources paired with lower-GI carbs like cruciferous veggies, squash, or leafy greens cooked in a healthy fat source like olive oil. A healthy breakfast would include things like whole eggs with leafy greens and avocado, loaded omelets, or smoked salmon on low-carb toast with avocado or cream cheese. A healthy lunch or dinner would include things like a salmon salad, chicken thighs with roasted squash and veggies, or a grilled steak with sautéed veggies. Before working out and between meals, you function best when snacking on healthy fats like nuts and seeds. After workouts, it's optimal to include a high-protein shake with fruit while keeping the fat intake low.

There are exceptions, but most Fat-Fueled Macro Types are naturally pear-shaped or apple-shaped and carry most of their weight in their lower half or torso. You may have been overweight for most of your life, or you may have come to a point where you stopped losing fat due to a medical condition. You tend to do better on lower-carb eating plans, but this does not mean you *need* to do a ketogenic diet. If your goal is weight loss and you have experienced any of these conditions, you most likely need to reduce carbs and increase fat.

This plan is excellent for those with a slower metabolism, moderately low carb tolerance, and/or slightly compromised hormonal function who are desperately trying to drop body fat in a way that doesn't make them feel like they are perpetually starving. This approach is higher in healthy fats, moderate in protein, and moderately low in carbs. While many people need this type of approach, it is not a well-defined diet niche because it is not extremely low fat, like what bodybuilders eat, and it's not extremely high fat, like the keto diet.

Think of *restored internal health* as the first priority, with fat loss as the second priority. If you are sick and tired of feeling exhausted, hungry, burnt out, and have absolutely no idea how to balance a plate, this nutrition plan is for you. You are at the point where you only know what *does not* work and have zero idea how to carve out a path that does. You may be experiencing perimenopause, you may have PCOS, you may be on medication for your hormones, or you may have prediabetes but do not want to commit to a ketogenic approach because you need something more sustainable.

This is also the plan for those seeking a feminine-yet-fit aesthetic who have zero interest in getting ripped or shredded. If you are a woman plateaued at over 30 percent body fat or a man plateaued at over 23 percent body fat and are looking to not only drop body fat but restore your health and finally feel better from the inside out, this approach is ideal.

LOW-CARB/HIGH-FAT PLANS

For people who are a Fat-Fueled Macro Type, the keto diet is extremely effective for fat loss. It is ideal for those with a very low carb tolerance who have trouble managing insulin properly; for others, it's a method you can try, but it won't necessarily be more effective than other programs. Be aware that it takes time for your body to switch from running on carbs to becoming truly fat-adapted, meaning you are creating ketones. Some people can become keto-adapted in a day or two; for others, it takes a week or two. During this transitional period, people commonly experience what's known as the *keto flu*, which is caused by an electrolyte imbalance that occurs when your insulin levels first drop.

This can give you headaches and leave you feeling nauseated and dizzy at first. You can navigate this electrolyte imbalance by adding more salt to your food (five times the recommended daily allowance). It may sound like a *ton* of salt, but you are excreting it way faster than normal, so it won't accumulate in your body.

This is not a quick fix but more of a lifestyle change. Consistency is a major factor for success with the ketogenic approach. If you exceed your carb intake on this plan, you will kick your body out of ketosis, and you'll need to become fat-adapted again. If you go off-track with this style of eating, you need to do so in a way that keeps you in a state of ketosis; for instance, eating higher calories but at keto ratios, with more healthy fats and protein, not more carbs.

People ask me all the time if they can "lose weight faster on keto." It depends. For some, it's a hard *yes*. If you are someone who has very low carb tolerance and simply cannot lose weight on a carb-inclusive nutrition plan due to insulin management issues, it will absolutely help you. This is a wonderful approach for those with type 2 diabetes, prediabetes, insulin resistance, PCOS, and hormone imbalances.

When other macro types follow a keto diet, they may lose weight faster at first due to water weight, but this does not mean they are going to lose actual stored body fat faster than they would with a more carb-heavy diet. And if you truly want to maximize the benefits of the ketogenic approach, you have to ask yourself if you are willing to commit to this as a lifestyle for a minimum of three to six months.

Many people ask if it is possible to go lower in carbs and higher in fats but not to the same extremes as keto. The answer also is *yes*. If you are trying to fine-tune your body fat percentage to below 15 to 20 percent for a woman or below 10 percent for a man, a low-carb/high-fat approach is going to be less targeted than a high-protein/low-fat method or a ketogenic method. Even so, a low-carb/high-fat diet has immense value.

TYPE 5: FAT-FUELED/LOW-CARB MACRO TYPE

If you fit the Fat-Fueled/Low-Carb Macro Type, you function best when a larger portion of your calories comes from fats. An ideal eating plan for this macro type consists of 75 percent fat, 20 percent protein, and 5 percent carbs. Of the three macronutrients, you do best when you consume a higher proportion of your total daily caloric intake from fat, with moderate protein and very low carb intake.

Typical meals for the Fat-Fueled/Low-Carb Macro Type will have your portions looking oddly smaller due to the caloric density of high-fat foods. With an emphasis on dietary fat, over 75 percent of the food on your plate will be from healthy fats, with moderate protein and your carbs coming from low-GI sources like leafy greens, cruciferous veggies, squash, or low-sugar fruit. A healthy breakfast would include things like whole eggs with bacon and a side of spinach sautéed in olive or coconut oil, chicken sausage with avocado and a whole egg with a side of mixed greens, or a frittata. A healthy lunch or dinner would include things like a salad topped with healthy fats with a small piece of salmon or grass-fed steak, chicken thighs with sautéed veggies, or a spaghetti squash casserole loaded with healthy fats. Before a workout and between meals, you function best when snacking on healthy fats like nuts and seeds. After workouts, it's optimal to include a high-protein shake with low-sugar fruit while keeping the fat intake low.

Fats provide an alternative form of functional energy, which is especially helpful for those who can't properly process carbohydrates. When your body struggles to handle carbs, you will experience compromised energy levels no matter how many carbs you consume. If this is you, you most likely are experiencing more serious medical issues such as insulin resistance, prediabetes, diabetes, PCOS, or other hormonal imbalances. You have probably struggled with weight loss, trying other extreme diet approaches that included higher levels of carbs only to find them frustratingly ineffective. It may seem to you that you cannot drop body fat no matter what you do. You are frustrated because your body in no way, shape, or form reflects your sincere efforts to improve your health. You gain weight so easily and lose it so slowly that attempting to sustain any type of plan leaves you feeling so frustrated that you no longer even want to try. You experience sugar cravings on a regular basis to the point that it is very hard for you to feel satisfied at the end of a meal. No matter how much sugar you eat, you are left wanting more and more and more.

If this sounds like your experience, the first thing I want you to know is that you are not crazy, you are not insane, and your feelings are 100 percent justified because your body is biochemically starving on a cellular level. This means that the carbs you *do* eat are not being used by your body as fuel due to insulin resistance. Your cells never receive the energy from the food you are consuming, so even though you are eating, you are not able to access the energy that food is supposed to give you. To make matters even worse, your body is in a perpetual state of retaining fat, making it impossible for you to tap into your stored body fat for energy either. This is why shifting your eating away from carbs will serve as the ultimate game-changer for you. Your body will be able to tap into fat as the fuel source with absolute ease because there will be no other option but to convert dietary fats into easily utilizable fuel.

When you think of eating for the Fat-Fueled/Low-Carb Macro Type, think of *fat-loss breakthrough*. When you align yourself with a nutrition style that enables your body to function the way it was always meant to, it's like finding the love of your life after years of misery with someone who just didn't get you. Imagine being able to enjoy days filled with energy, without sugar cravings; and when you expend effort exercising, you are no longer spinning your wheels and getting absolutely nowhere. You are burning fat and feeling great!

This approach is a high-fat, moderate-protein, and very-low-carb approach to nutrition, which is commonly referred to as the ketogenic diet. It has this name because the body is no longer fueled by carbs; it is fueled by healthy fats that generate ketones as the primary energy source. This allows the body to utilize fat as a fuel source and is a great method for those with the lowest carb tolerance levels. This approach is wonderful for those who need a simple and straightforward way to drop body fat. This is also great for those who thrive on well-defined boundaries, finding it easier to stay on track when there are more rigid guidelines of what you can and cannot eat. If you are a woman over 35 percent body fat or a man over 30 percent body fat and need a simple yet effective approach to begin the fat-loss journey, this is a great place to start.

WHAT IF YOU WANT TO TRY KETO, BUT IT ISN'T YOUR MACRO TYPE?

While a high-fat diet, like keto, is ideal for the Fat-Fueled Macro Type and anyone with certain conditions like diabetes or PCOS, this does not mean that other macro types can't benefit from a fat-dominant approach. In 2016 and 2017, I tried the keto diet to gain a better understanding of it so I could best guide my clients. Although I do not have any of the medical issues listed that would make me the Fat-Fueled Macro Type, I found that I was still able to get results on the keto diet. While I stopped eating this way because it was ultimately unsustainable for me, I enjoyed the food, the energy, and mental clarity and appreciated the feeling of fullness from eating more fats. But I didn't need to remove carbs from my diet to lose weight.

If you, like me, don't have any specific medical reason to go very low-carb, you can still try a keto diet. Just keep in mind that because it can be a more restrictive meal plan, it is likely going to be a temporary solution, and you may end up transitioning to a higher-carbs approach eventually. Following this style of eating is great for a three- to six-month period to reverse carb tolerance issues, but it is not something you ought to plan to sustain for life if you don't have a valid medical reason to do so.

· · ·

Now that you know your macro type and its corresponding nutrient ratios, it's time to get into the nitty-gritty of your plan: what you will eat, how much, and when.

6

Setting Up Your Plan

The most important part of designing a healthy program is start-ing with a clear vision of what success will look like for you. This means knowing your current body fat percentage and defining a healthy, sustainable target body composition.

You may have an image in your mind of what you would like to look like. Maybe you have pictures on your phone of your favorite celebrity or influencer and want to push yourself to their level. Maybe you long to fit into your prepregnancy clothes again. Maybe your health has been declining for years, and you fear that if you don't do something about it now, you'll end up like family members who've neglected their health and lost years and quality of life as a result. Maybe you just want to keep the lights on when you have sex with your partner and not feel self-conscious.

To turn your vision of success into an actionable plan, we first must translate your current state of health to a rough body fat percentage. You can get an exact number by having a professional run a test on your body composition, but you can also estimate it by sight. A self-assessment is more than sufficient to gauge your starting point. Use the visual chart below to estimate your current body composition.[1]

You will most likely fall into one of four categories, depending on where you are in your health journey:

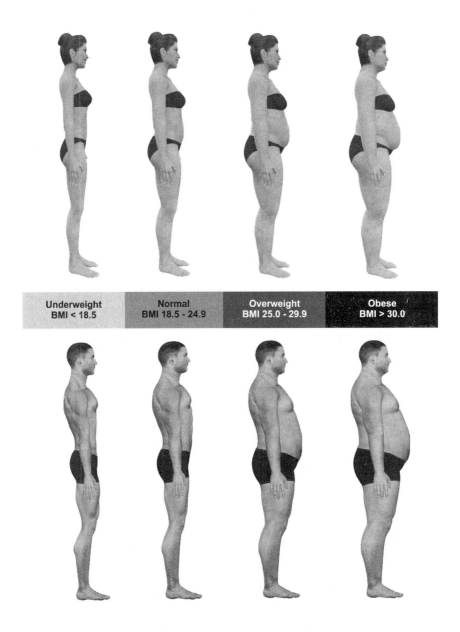

© Levi Bunnell

OBESE (MORE THAN 50 POUNDS TO LOSE) If this is you, remember that you don't need to make a lot of changes at once. When you have more weight to lose, you can see progress by making positive changes relative to your current lifestyle, not necessarily trying an aggressive program. For example, if you are used to eating upwards of 3,000 calories per day, living a sedentary lifestyle, and drinking wine every day, you don't need to adopt a radical exercise and nutrition regimen to see a change in your health. When you're getting started, simple changes like cutting out alcohol, going on daily walks, and cutting back on processed foods will be enough. In terms of progress, there is a lot of low-hanging fruit under these circumstances, which will only require a modest effort on your part to see a significant improvement.

OVERWEIGHT (25 TO 50 POUNDS TO LOSE) Whether you became overweight in recent months or it crept up on you over the years, it will take a more conscious effort for you to lose weight at this stage. This is most true for women and men over 35 years old, as hormonal and metabolic factors make it more challenging to drop body fat. This means small changes such as walking, cutting out alcohol, and reducing sugar intake won't be enough if you have a time-sensitive fat-loss goal, even if they are great lifestyle changes. To make great progress and fast, you'll have to set specific macro goals and stay within a 10 percent margin of error following them.

UNLOCKING YOUR MACRO TYPE: REAL STORIES, REAL SUCCESSES

Alva, Protein-Fueled Macro Type

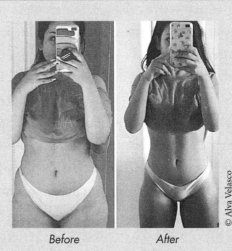

Before   *After*

Alva is a pear-shaped endomorph, and she is a perfect example of why I wrote this book. Most people assume that endomorphs need to go lower in carbs. Although Alva is an endomorph, she doesn't have a low carb tolerance, and she was able to lose weight with consistent nutrition and workouts. Her calorie intake ranged from 1,200 to 1,500 over the course of her program with adjustments made weekly to support her progress. It took her approximately six months to reach her goal physique for her petite 5-foot, 1-inch frame, and then she went on to maintenance eating over 2,000 calories a day.

NORMAL WEIGHT (0 TO 25 POUNDS TO LOSE) If you fall into this category, you may have friends and family who say you look "fine" and don't need to lose any weight. Still, you want to look and feel more fit, with defined muscles and a flatter stomach. Maybe you feel like your energy isn't what it used to be, or you wish you could fit into those favorite jeans from a few years ago. The closer you get to your goals and the less weight you have to lose, the more exacting you need to be with your macros. For maximum results, you will need to follow your nutrition protocol within a much tighter margin of error, around 5 percent.

UNDERWEIGHT (NEED TO GAIN WEIGHT) While this isn't as common, many people struggle to gain weight. It can be just as challenging to add quality weight as it can be to lose fat. If this is you, you will need to follow your nutrition protocol with as much intention as possible, because macros have a huge impact on the quality of the weight you gain. Far too many people take the "eat everything" approach to weight gain, which may raise the number on the scale but won't give you the kind of healthy, shapely, and strong physique you're after.

Quality weight gain comes from gaining lean muscle mass without gaining body fat. This is only possible when you consume the correct macros for lean muscle gain. Without a targeted approach, you may gain weight, but most of that weight will be fat.

Whatever your starting point, beginning your plan is where the magic happens. This is where your dreams become goals, and those goals become an actionable strategy. Once you master that strategy, you can't help but see results. It's not a question of *if* you will reach your goals but *when*. Now that you know where you're starting from, it's time to set goals.

Setting Your Goal

The main goals to choose from when approaching your body composition are fat loss, muscle gain, or maintenance. Once you set your goal, we will break down the mechanics of calculating your caloric intake and macronutrient ratios so you can create a specific and detailed vision of what success looks like for you.

But first, we need to have a frank discussion about how long this process will take and what results are possible. I've found over the years that people tend to be impatient with the process of fat loss and often have unrealistic expectations. A realistic goal is foundational for success. All too often, people think they aren't making progress and feel discouraged, when in fact they are improving at the fastest possible rate for healthy, sustainable results.

Everyone reading this can make measurable improvements. For fat loss, the maximum rate of progress a female can expect when adhering 100 percent to a nutrition and training plan designed to lose 1 pound of fat per week is a decrease of about 0.5 percent body fat per week. The absolute maximum rate of fat loss a female can attain naturally is a drop of 0.8 percent body fat per week (this is the rate I use to develop protocols for fitness competitors). It is impractical to expect to lose fat any faster than this rate in a manner that doesn't incorporate steroids or surgery. That said, let's make sure your current body fat percentage and your goal body fat percentage are in line with reality.

A common goal for most women and men is to lose the belly. You don't want to get ripped, but you want to look and feel healthier. If you are a woman with a waist measurement of over 35 inches (or a male over 40 inches), you are at risk for several diseases due to high levels of visceral fat. In this case, a practical goal is to drop your visceral fat and bring your waist measurement to less than 30 inches for women (or 36 inches for men).

If you don't have an accurate way to monitor your body fat percentage (most people don't), it's more practical to set a goal based on your torso measurement. In my work with over 40,000 clients over the last decade, I've found 80 to 90 percent of people can lower their waist measurement by a maximum of ½ inch per week when 100 percent on track with nutrition and training. With clients who adhered to their nutrition and training plans 70 to 80 percent of the time, I found most were able to progress at a rate of ¼ inch lost per week. So if your goal is to go from a 35-inch waist to a 30-inch waist, it will take ten weeks (at an average rate of ½ inch lost per week) to twenty weeks (at an average rate of ¼ inch lost per week). This means the entire process will take three to six months' time, a much longer journey than most expect. Keep these calculations in mind when gauging your own journey. Be patient, be consistent, and you'll get the best outcome!

If you are a woman and want a six-pack, you will need to be around 13 percent body fat or less. Or maybe you don't aspire to have visible abs but want to drop your lower-belly pooch that seems to *never* go away. In reality, it's not that low-belly fat never goes away, it's that you haven't dropped your body fat percentage low enough to facilitate a noticeable change in that area.

Let's say you are 30 percent body fat and have spent one month working hard to stick to the nutrition plan for your macro type. Now, at 28 percent body fat, you're frustrated. All you see is your stomach. You ask me, "Christine, why haven't I lost my lower stomach yet? What exercise can I do to get rid of my belly?"

I review your progress and see that you've dropped 2 percent body fat in a month, have taken 2 inches off your waist, and have made a serious overhaul of your eating habits. My friend, you've done incredibly well! You still see fat on your lower belly because your body fat isn't low enough yet for the result you're looking for. It will get there.

Most women don't begin to see their torsos completely flatten until they've dropped to at least 23 percent body fat. In our example, this means if you can continue sustaining 0.5 percent body fat loss per week, going from 28 to 23 percent body fat will take ten weeks, or another two and a half months.

The bottom line is, it takes longer than you may think to reach your goal. If you feel like your progress is slow, it does not mean you are doing anything wrong; it means that you need to keep going. Quitting won't get you there faster. And there aren't any shortcuts that will get you there either.

Now that you have prepared your mind, emotions, and body to start your journey, let's set up your plan!

1. DETERMINING BASAL METABOLIC RATE

The number of calories your body needs to function is called your *basal metabolic rate,* or BMR. This value tells you how much energy you need to sustain your current body mass, assuming you are at rest and expending zero physical energy. You can have professionals measure this value, or you can calculate it using the Mifflin-St Jeor equations, a model that uses age, height, and weight to estimate BMR. Hospitals and nutrition clinics use these equations to determine the calorie requirements of their patients. (There are four BMR equations with widespread use, but the Mifflin-St Jeor equations tend to yield the most reliable results.) The Mifflin-St Jeor equations are:

Female: BMR = (4.536 × weight in pounds) + (15.88 × height in inches) − (5 × age in years) − 16

Male: BMR = (4.536 × weight in pounds) + (15.88 × height in inches) − (5 × age in years) + 5

For example, a 35-year-old female who is 5 feet, 5 inches and 175 pounds:

$$BMR = (4.536 \times \textbf{175 pounds}) + (15.88 \times \textbf{65 inches})$$
$$- (5 \times \textbf{35 years}) - 161$$
$$BMR = (793.8) + (1032.2) - (175) - 161$$
$$BMR = 1,490 \text{ calories}$$

2. DETERMINING ACTIVITY FACTOR

Using your BMR with your activity level, you can calculate how many calories your body needs to meet your daily energy expenditure needs based on your daily activity levels. Be honest with yourself about your current level of activity. The following activity factors (abbreviated as AF below) reflect different levels of activity in an average week:

- If you are sedentary and do not exercise, your AF is 1.2.
- If you exercise lightly 1 to 3 times per week, your AF is 1.375.
- If you exercise 3 to 4 times per week, your AF is 1.4.
- If you exercise 4 to 5 times per week, your AF is 1.55.
- If you exercise 5 to 6 times per week, your AF is 1.65.
- If you exercise 6 or 7 times per week, your AF is 1.725.
- If you exercise 7 times per week and have a physically demanding job, your AF is 1.9.

So a woman who has a sedentary job and works out three to four times a week has an activity factor of 1.375. While she does work out, the fact that she is sedentary most of the time pushes her into a lower range. It's always better to underestimate the activity factor.

3. DETERMINING TOTAL DAILY ENERGY EXPENDITURE

Your total daily energy expenditure (TDEE) is the number of calories you need to sustain your current body mass, factoring in the calories you burn through activity. We determine the TDEE by multiplying the BMR with the activity factor.

Example: A 35-year-old female who is 5 feet, 5 inches and 175 pounds and has a BMR of 1,490 and an activity factor of 1.375 yields the following total daily energy expenditure:

$$TDEE = BMR \times activity\ factor$$
$$TDEE = 1,490 \times 1.375$$
$$TDEE = 2,048.75$$

4. DETERMINING TARGET CALORIC INTAKE

The next step is to determine your target caloric intake, which depends on your goal. If you want to lose fat, you subtract 500 from your TDEE to get your target caloric intake. To gain weight, you add 500 to your TDEE. To maintain your current weight, your TDEE is your target caloric intake. So, depending on your goal, you should change your caloric intake as follows:

Fat-loss caloric intake (for 1 lb of fat loss/week) = TDEE − 500

Maintenance caloric intake = TDEE − 0

Weight-gain caloric intake (for 1 lb of mass gain/week) = TDEE + 500

For example, a 35-year-old female who is 5 feet, 5 inches and 175 pounds, has a TDEE of 2,048.75, and wants to lose 1 pound of body fat per week needs the following target caloric intake:

Fat-loss caloric intake = TDEE − 500
Fat-loss caloric intake = 2,048.75 − 500
Fat-loss caloric intake = 1,548.75 (rounded to 1,549)

5. APPLYING THE MACRONUTRIENT RATIOS FOR EACH MACRO TYPE

Now you are going to factor in your macro type to get your appropriate daily macronutrient intake. Calculate this by multiplying your daily caloric intake by your target macronutrient percentages for each macro (proteins, carbs, and fats). (And remember that if you want to lose body fat, you'll need to be in a suitable *caloric deficit,* or these recommendations will not matter, even if your *macro ratios* are perfect. Only when your calories are at the correct level will changing your proportions of fats, carbs, and proteins drive progress.)

This means you take your target caloric intake (e.g., 1,549 calories) and multiply it by the percentages of each macro to get the daily calories you need for each. (So for, say, 39 percent, you would multiply by 0.39.) You then take the daily calorie amount for each macro and divide it by the calories per gram of that nutrient to get the number of grams of each macro you should consume each day.

MACRO TYPE	% CARBS	% PROTEIN	% FAT
CARB-FUELED	45.0	30.0	25.0
PROTEIN-FUELED	32.5	39.0	28.5
PROTEIN-FUELED / LOW CARB	26.5	37.5	36.0
FAT-FUELED	17.5	27.5	55.0
FAT-FUELED / LOW CARB	5.0	20.0	75.0
USDA	60.0	10.0	30.0

For example, a 35-year-old female who is 5 feet, 5 inches and 175 pounds, with a TDEE of 2,049, and who is looking to lose 1 pound of body fat per week, has a target intake of 1,549 calories. If she is a Protein-Fueled Macro Type (see above) and has a moderate carb tolerance, she would need to set up her macros as follows:

39% Protein: 0.39 × 1,549 = 604.1 calories from protein

604.1 cal ÷ 4 cal per g protein = **151 g protein each day**

28.5% Fats: 0.285 × 1,549 = 441.5 calories from fat

441.5 cal ÷ 9 cal per g fat = **49.1 g fats each day**

32.5% Carbs: 0.325 × 1,549 = 503.4 calories from carbs

503.4 calories ÷ 4 cal per g carbs =

125.9 g carbs each day

Now It's Your Turn

Hopefully, the plan is starting to click in your mind — you've now determined which macro type fits you best, you have your target daily calorie intake, and you've used that info to determine your macronutrient goals for each day. Now that you've seen how this works in the example, it's time for you to plug in your personal values.

1. DETERMINE YOUR BASAL METABOLIC RATE

Female: BMR = (4.536 × weight in pounds) +

(15.88 × height in inches) − (5 × age in years) − 161

My BMR = (4.536 × _____ **lbs**) + (15.88 × _____ **in**) − (5 × _____ **yrs**) − 161

BMR = (_____) + (_____) − (_____) − 161 = _____

Male: BMR = (4.536 × weight in pounds) +

(15.88 × height in inches) − (5 × age in years) + 5

My BMR = (4.536 × _____ **lbs**) + (15.88 × _____ **in**) − (5 × _____ **yrs**) + 5

BMR = (_____) + (_____) − (_____) + 5 = _____

My BMR = _____ calories

2. DETERMINE YOUR ACTIVITY FACTOR

- If you are sedentary and do not exercise, your AF is 1.2.
- If you exercise lightly 1 to 3 times per week, your AF is 1.375.
- If you exercise 3 to 4 times per week, your AF is 1.4.
- If you exercise 4 to 5 times per week, your AF is 1.55.
- If you exercise 5 to 6 times per week, your AF is 1.65.
- If you exercise 6 or 7 times per week, your AF is 1.725.
- If you exercise 7 times per week and have a physically demanding job, your AF is 1.9.

My activity factor = _____

3. DETERMINE YOUR TOTAL DAILY ENERGY EXPENDITURE

TDEE = BMR × activity factor

TDEE = _____ × _____ = _____

My TDEE = _____

4. DETERMINE YOUR TARGET CALORIC INTAKE

Fat-loss caloric intake (for 1 lb of fat loss/week) = TDEE – 500

Maintenance caloric intake = TDEE – 0

Weight-gain caloric intake (for 1 lb of mass gain/week) = TDEE + 500

Calculate your target caloric intake according to your goal:

Fat-loss caloric intake = _____ (TDEE) – 500 = _____

Maintenance caloric intake: _____ (TDEE) – 0 = _____

Weight-gain caloric intake= _____ (TDEE) + 500 = _____

My target caloric intake = _____

5. APPLY THE MACRONUTRIENT RATIOS FOR YOUR MACRO TYPE

MACRO TYPE	% CARBS	% PROTEIN	% FAT
CARB-FUELED	45.0	30.0	25.0
PROTEIN-FUELED	32.5	39.0	28.5
PROTEIN-FUELED / LOW CARB	26.5	37.5	36.0
FAT-FUELED	17.5	27.5	55.0
FAT-FUELED / LOW CARB	5.0	20.0	75.0
USDA	60.0	10.0	30.0

_____% **protein** (from chart): _____

(**% protein** ÷ 100) _____ × (target caloric intake) _____ = _____ calories from protein

_____ calories from protein ÷ 4 cal per g protein = _____ **g protein each day**

_____% **fat** (from chart): _____

(**% fat** ÷ 100) _____ × (target caloric intake) _____ = _____ calories from fat _____

calories from fat ÷ 9 cal per g fat = _____ **g fats each day**

_____% **carbs** (from chart): _____

(**% carbs** ÷ 100) _____ × (target caloric intake) _____ = _____ calories from carbs

_____ calories from carbs ÷ 4 cal per g carbs = _____ **g carbs each day**

6. APPLY A TRAINING PLAN FOR YOUR MACRO TYPE

While 80 to 90 percent of your progress will come from targeted nutrition, proper training methods also are essential to your overall success. Most of what I've shared with you so far has been related to the individual macronutrients and fat loss. However, when it comes to changing your body composition, it's not only about losing fat; it's also about gaining muscle. (See Chapter 9 for all the details on how to train according to your macro type.)

Let me show you how this will maximize your results. You can lose 1 pound of body fat per week by setting up a caloric deficit of 500 calories per day. When it comes to gaining muscle mass, the average man can gain about 2 to 4 pounds of muscle per month, where a woman can gain about 1 to 2 pounds of muscle. The muscle tissue that you build through exercise will increase the number of calories you use all day, every day, not just while you're working out. In this way, you can lose more fat *faster* than if you're only eating for your macro type.

Now, like diet, muscle gain is not just a function of going through the motions of a one-size-fits-all regimen. Optimal training volume and intensity are affected by variables such as genetics, hormone levels, and rest. This is all to say that the training method you choose must be a match for your dominant macro type.

Each macro type encompasses various ranges of adaptability when it comes to body composition. The carb-fueled type has the easiest time dropping fat but struggles the hardest to gain muscle. The protein-fueled type can lose fat with ease, but it's not as effortless as those who are carb dominant. Protein-fueled types can experience faster muscle gains compared to those who are carb-fueled. Fat-fueled individuals tend to struggle with fat loss the most but gain muscle with ease and don't need to lift as heavy to experience great physical shifts. See detailed guidelines in Chapter 9 for training guidelines for your macro type, and create your customized targeted workout regime.

Planning Meals: What You Will Eat in a Day

Once you have your customized macronutrient targets and daily caloric intake goal, your objective is to eat whatever you want within those limits. It doesn't matter what you eat to add up to the right macro ratios, so long as you're hitting your target grams of proteins, carbs, and fats for the day.

If you are new to macros, this can be overwhelming, so I'm going to make it as easy as possible by providing simple guidelines of what a full day of eating would look like according to your macro type. This is ideal if you are overwhelmed by the concept of adding numbers and math to food. Keep in mind that there are infinite ways you could arrange your daily food intake and still hit your macro goals for the day. However, sometimes too much flexibility isn't ideal because it leaves too many options on the table when what you need is focused direction to get started so you know what foods to pick up at the grocery store. By breaking down your recommended macro type into examples of real whole foods instead of just numbers, you can more easily grasp what your meals should look like compared to how you are currently eating.

To begin, we need to understand which macronutrient categories real whole foods fall under. If you are new to macros, there's a bit of a learning curve here. If you are a Protein-Fueled Macro Type, you'll need to learn which foods are higher in protein. If you need to be lower in carb consumption, you should have a better idea of which foods you need to eat in small amounts. If you are a Fat-Fueled Macro Type, you need to know which foods support that. The problem is that real foods aren't always made up of one single macronutrient (although some are). For example, most think of eggs as "protein," but in reality, a single whole egg is 6.5 grams of protein and 5 grams of fat. In another example, it's obvious that bread is a carb, but so is broccoli. For this reason, refining how we view real whole foods in terms of macronutrients deserves a brief discussion.

While there are three macronutrients, when it comes to planning meals, I look at food in six categories, not three: lean proteins, fatty proteins, low-GI carbs, high-GI carbs, healthy fats, and fatty low-GI carbs.

LEAN PROTEIN

Chicken, egg whites, fish, turkey, lean beef, whey, collagen, etc.

I've split proteins into two categories based on their relative fat content. When you hear the term *lean protein*, think low fat. If you don't consider the fat content of your protein sources, you could easily overshoot your daily fat intake because there are a lot of proteins with a substantial portion of their calories from dietary fats. Again, fats are not "bad"; it's more a matter of ensuring you stay within your specific daily targets. I consider any protein with less than 10 grams of fat per serving (assuming you are getting at least 25 grams of protein per serving) to be a "lean" protein source. This is where foods like boneless skinless chicken breast, white fish, tuna, turkey, lean beef, protein powders, and egg whites tend to be excellent staples to ensure you are reaching your daily protein goal without overshooting your fat intake.

FATTY PROTEIN

Salmon, whole eggs, pork, rib eye, duck, lamb, etc.

Fatty-protein recipes tend to be tastier and may feel more like "regular food" to you if you aren't used to macro-based cooking. However, it is important to acknowledge that these contain greater amounts of fat, and as a result they should be carefully considered. Remember that you can eat whatever you wish as long as it fits your macros; however, if you are a Protein-Fueled Macro Type, you may find that if you consume fatty proteins with every meal (for example, whole eggs for breakfast, salmon for lunch, and duck for dinner) you will most likely go over your daily fat budget. Likewise, if you are a Fat-Fueled Macro Type, you need to be selecting *more* fatty protein sources as opposed to lean proteins. Instead of egg whites (which is common to a lot of bodybuilder-style meal plans), you would do better with fattier proteins like whole eggs. Remember to not overcomplicate this section. I consider a protein source to be "fatty" if it has *more* than 10 grams of fat per serving (assuming each serving contains roughly 20 to 25 grams of protein). This is where foods like fattier cuts of fish such as salmon, mackerel, trout, and albacore tuna are excellent food choices. In addition, think chicken thighs with the skin on, whole eggs, rib eye, duck, lamb, or hemp tofu as food options that are high in protein while providing a good source of dietary fats.

HIGH-GI CARBS
Rice, whole grains, oats, pasta, potatoes, banana, etc.

Carbs are broken down based on their ranking according to the glycemic index (GI) scale. This scale describes how quickly a given carbohydrate will increase your blood glucose level. If a carb is higher on the GI scale, it means it is converted to usable energy quickly, which is great as your body demands that energy if you are about to work out, play intense sports, or if you struggle to gain weight. However, if you are relatively sedentary, too much from this category of foods can lead to fat gain. Tracking high-GI carbs will be the biggest eye-opener for you if you have never tracked or portioned your foods before. This is because typical portion sizes at restaurants or even what you are used to preparing at home tend to be way larger than anything I will recommend here. As stated earlier, the USDA recommends 300 grams of carbs per day for adults and the WHO recommends 400 grams. Naturally, this would apply to only Carb-Fueled Macro Types who are also active; so it does not apply to most of us. Be prepared to recalibrate your mind, your eyes, and your plate. You will *not* starve on your new carb portions, but know that it will be an adjustment for the first week, as your body naturally detoxes from higher-carb foods that tend to include empty sugars. The body is great at acclimating, and it won't be long before you are feeling fuller sooner on a meal with a different macronutrient composition. If your macro type calls for high-GI carbs, you would do best with foods like bananas, rice, oats, potatoes, etc. as your carb sources.

LOW-GI CARBS

Leafy greens, veggies, mixed berries, squash, cruciferous veggies, etc.

Low-GI carbs are foods that are considered carbs based on their chemical composition, but they impact the body differently compared to high-GI carbs. When you consume them, they don't spike the blood sugar as high and, therefore, are a great alternative for those with insulin management issues. Low-GI carbs are foods that are higher in fiber and lower in sugar and that do not have a big impact on your insulin when consumed in moderate amounts (i.e., under about 10 to 15 grams of carbs per serving). This means incorporating nonstarchy green vegetables like asparagus, squash, leafy greens, low-sugar berries, and any other vegetable that doesn't cause a sharp insulin spike. Not only do low-GI carbs help you feel full and satisfied longer, but they also support weight loss by enabling you to keep your calories lower while consuming higher volumes of food.

FATTY LOW-GI CARBS

Low-carb high-fat bread, almond flour tortillas, coconut flour tortillas, veggies sautéed in healthy fats, veggie casseroles, cauliflower pizza crusts, healthy sauces/dips (i.e., hummus), coconut chips

You may be wondering what on earth are fatty low-GI carbs. These are foods that represent food items and preparation methods common to paleo, low-carb/high-fat, and keto diets. This means that the food is high in fat but low in carbs, but not so low in carbs that the carbs are insignificant. It's worth considering it a group especially for macro types 3 through 5, as these types of foods do become new staples in a real day of eating, and it's easier to organize how you eat around it.

Fatty low-GI carb recipes contain ingredients or foods that are high in fat and low in carbs. It can be something as simple as Brussels sprouts sautéed in at least 10 grams of olive oil. To be considered a fatty low-GI carb, there needs to be at least 10 grams of fat present in the serving, thereby making a significant source of dietary fat intake.

HEALTHY FATS

Olive oil, coconut oil, avocado oil, nuts, seeds, ghee, grass-fed butter, olives, walnuts, almonds, chia, flax, hemp

This is one of the simplest categories as these foods are primarily just fat, with a few of them having fiber, like avocado, nuts, and seeds. When incorporating a healthy fat into your meals as a stand-alone ingredient, it is typically part of the cooking method associated with the meal unless it's a topping on a salad or an addition to a shake. To be considered a healthy fat, the majority of the food needs to be fat. It will be eye-opening for most to see the caloric contribution of these foods, which are considered healthy. They are healthy, but the portions need to be carefully considered, as the calories add up quickly. If you need to consume lower amounts of dietary fats due to your macro type, you will find that you need to choose wisely so you don't overdo it in this category, which is one of the most common mistakes.

COUNTLESS FOODS

These items contain less than 3 grams of carbs per serving and typically contain fiber. Think of bell peppers, cucumbers, celery, leafy greens, and other low-calorie veggies, along with fresh herbs and a squeeze of lemon or lime. These foods add a trivial number of calories to your meals and allow you to boost the volume on your plate without spiking your insulin. The goal is to allow you to have mindless items you can freely consume without having to think, track, or stress when you are feeling like you want "more."

If you are feeling hungry, you can have the following foods at any time without having to count or track:

Kale	Dill pickles	Spices	Black coffee
Spinach	Banana peppers	Fresh herbs	Tea
Arugula	Hot peppers	Hot sauce	Sparkling water
Mixed greens	Vinegar	Lemons	Café Americano
Bell peppers	Onions	Limes	Stevia
Cucumbers	Garlic	Kimchi	Monk fruit

At-a-Glance Meal Guidelines

So how should you eat for your macro type? Think of these guidelines like the blueprints for a home. The fundamental structure of the home is already predesigned, but you have the flexibility to choose key attributes like the exterior colors, the shutters, the countertops, the tiles, the flooring, etc. Only in this case, you get to choose the type of lean protein when specified, the type of carbs, etc. The fundamental structure of how a full day of eating is organized varies based on your macro type.

These guidelines enable you to see the major distinctions between the macro types and how that translates to the types of food you should put on your plate.

I've broken down a full day of eating parameters based on estimated portions you should be consuming of the different real food-based macronutrient categories. Inside each food category, you'll be able to choose among several foods. The great news is that you get to choose your foods, providing limitless options and tons of food freedom for every macro type. Keep in mind that the exact detailed portions in the plans outlined below will vary based on your specific target caloric intake; however, this is a great reference point to start assembling a full day of eating. For specific sample meal plans and recipes for each macro type, turn to pages 160 and 194.

CARB-FUELED MACRO TYPE

You will want to organize your plate for breakfast, lunch, and dinner to include this type of breakdown:

    4 to 6 oz lean proteins
    8 to 10 oz high-GI carbs
    2 to 4 oz low-GI carbs
    <0.5 oz healthy fats

Prior to workouts include:
    4 oz high-GI carbs

After workouts include:
    4 to 6 oz lean proteins (or 1 scoop of a protein supplement)
    4 oz high-GI carbs

Snacks:
    >4 oz high-GI carbs

PROTEIN-FUELED MACRO TYPE

You will want to organize your plate for breakfast, lunch, and dinner to include this type of breakdown:

4 to 6 oz lean proteins
<4 oz high-GI carbs
2 to 4 oz low-GI carbs
<0.5 oz healthy fats

Prior to workouts include:
2 oz high-GI carbs

After workouts include:
4- to 6 oz lean proteins (or 1 scoop of a protein supplement)
2 oz high-GI carbs

Snacks:
4 to 6 oz lean proteins (or 1 scoop of a protein supplement)

PROTEIN-FUELED/LOW-CARB MACRO TYPE

You will want to organize your plate for breakfast, lunch, and dinner to include this type of breakdown:

4 oz fatty proteins
2 to 4 oz high-GI carbs
4 to 6 oz low-GI carbs
0.5 to 1 oz healthy fats

Prior to workouts include:
2 oz high-GI carbs

After workouts include:
4 to 6 oz lean proteins (or 1 scoop of a protein supplement)
2 oz high-GI carbs

Snacks:
4 to 6 oz fatty proteins

FAT-FUELED MACRO TYPE

You will want to organize your plate for breakfast, lunch, and dinner to include this type of breakdown:

4 oz fatty proteins

2 to 4 oz high-GI carbs (you are to keep this portion to only one of the three major meals; it is advised to include with breakfast and omit for lunch and dinner)

4 to 6 oz low-GI carbs

0.5 to 1 oz healthy fats

Prior to workouts include:

2 oz high-GI carbs

After workouts include:

4 to 6 oz lean proteins (or 1 scoop of a protein supplement)

2 oz high-GI carbs

Snacks:

Keep snacking to a minimum and focus on countless foods (see page 152)

FAT-FUELED/LOW-CARB MACRO TYPE

You will want to organize your plate for breakfast, lunch, and dinner to include this type of breakdown:

3 oz fatty proteins
<4 oz low-GI carbs
>1 oz healthy fats

Prior to workouts include:
3 oz fatty proteins

After workouts include:
4 to 6 oz lean proteins (or 1 scoop of a protein supplement)
2 oz low-GI carbs

Snacks:
1 oz healthy fats

. . .

Now that you have your plan and understand the science behind it, you're almost set to take off on your body transformation journey. But first, let's take a look at what this means in your day-to-day life with some more detailed meal plans for each macro type.

7

Eating for Each Macro Type and Sample Meal Plans

The ultimate challenge for most people starting a macros program is relearning how to eat. This is a difficult concept, as we all have deep-seated ideas about eating that we have acquired over the years, stemming from our upbringing, culture, and preferences.

Unfortunately for most, the way of eating you are used to tends to be out of alignment with your optimal nutrition. I've seen this happen countless times with my clients. They will question all of my recommendations and convince themselves that this new way of eating is so different, there is no way they could stick to it. Yet, after a few days, they find themselves feeling better than ever. Their energy levels are higher, their skin is clearer, they're experiencing less bloating and sugar cravings, and their digestion has improved. After a few weeks, their clothes are fitting better or even getting looser, and they're seeing and feeling things change in their bodies that they thought were impossible. When relearning how to eat, it's important to remember that you are going to experience a physical and emotional recalibration. Huh? Let me explain.

Most people eat until they feel emotionally satisfied, physically stuffed, or both. Before you commit to making a conscious effort to eat healthy, you are most likely eating whatever is most convenient, affordable, and satisfying in the moment. This doesn't account for your body's legitimate nutrient needs.

Depending on your macro type, you may find that you need much more of the dominant macronutrient than you're used to eating. Let's take a look at these macro-type eating styles and sample meal plans.

Type 1: Carb-Fueled Macro Type

SAMPLE 2,000-CALORIE MEAL PLAN

30% Protein | 45% Carbs | 25% Fats

Overview

Most carb-fueled nutrition plans are for people who have a hard time gaining weight (aka ectomorphs) or are seeking to add lean muscle. These plans have a higher volume of carbs per meal and higher-carb snacks. Carb-fueled plans tend to include a caloric intake for body weight maintenance (at the minimum) or a caloric surplus. For those looking to gain lean muscle mass, I recommend adding 300 calories to their TDEE (total daily energy expenditure). For those seeking to gain weight overall, I recommend adding a maximum of 500 calories to their TDEE. For women, this type of plan tends to start no lower than 1,700 to 1,800 calories, and for men at 2,000 to 2,200 calories. Remember, depending on how active you are, these meal plans can easily be in the range of 3,000 to 5,000 calories.

Pre-Workout Nutrition

If you are training first thing in the morning, I advise getting at least 25 grams of carbs pre-workout. If you work out later in the day, your last meal can serve as your pre-workout meal.

Post-Workout Nutrition

I advise consuming at least 25 grams of protein and at least 10 grams of carbs post-workout. It's important to keep the fat content very low in your post-workout meal so as not to slow down your body's absorption of proteins, which support muscle recovery, and carbs, which support glycogen replenishment.

Meal Timing

When eating according to a higher-carb protocol, you will get full pretty fast. You may find yourself complaining about all the carbs you need to eat. If you do so in front of me, I will roll my eyes at you, LOL. A lot of people would *love* to need to eat more carbs. In most cases, since you already have a high tolerance for carbs, I don't advise intermittent fasting. You may need some breathing room between meals to digest your food before you have to eat again. I recommend eating three meals and three snacks: a pre-workout snack, a post-workout snack, and a third snack. You are welcome to condense the meals, but most people find it difficult to eat that much in one sitting and enjoy a more spread-out meal schedule to avoid getting super full. I suggest waiting at least 2 hours between meals, with the exception of your post-workout meal. You are welcome to eat your next meal right after a post-workout shake if that works for you. For example, if you hit the gym in the early morning, you would eat a snack before the gym, then drink a post-workout shake within 30 minutes after working out. After that, you don't need to wait to eat breakfast.

Snacks

Between meals, it is best to keep your snacks high in quality carbohydrates. This means choosing whole foods high in micronutrients, antioxidants, and fiber. Fresh fruit, veggies, and whole grains are excellent snacks for the Carb-Fueled Macro Type. For those struggling to hit their carb macros, the best choices are nutrient-dense foods like rice cakes, bananas, coconut water, grapes, toast with jelly, dried fruit, oats, and fruit smoothies. If you find the carb portions in your meals too big for your liking, you can reduce the size of your meals and eat some of the carbs between meals as snacks.

The Plan

The chart that follows outlines a sample meal plan broken down into a full day of eating for a Carb-Fueled Macro Type. The target daily caloric intake for this meal plan is 2,000 calories at 30 percent protein, 45 percent carbs, and 25 percent fat.

The menu is broken down into pre- and post-workout meals, breakfast, lunch, dinner, and snacks. It is written as though you are working out first thing in the morning. If you work out at a different time of day, simply move the pre- and post-workout meals accordingly.

Each meal is broken down into each food, quantity, and macronutrient per line. It is organized in this manner so you can see precisely how each food contributes to each meal, as well as the bigger picture of the entire day. This is particularly useful in making substitutions, so you know exactly how much of each macronutrient you need to substitute. You will notice that the meals tend to be higher in carbs, moderate in protein, and lower in dietary fats.

At the bottom of the chart, you will see the daily totals of calories, carbs, fiber, fat, and protein intake compared to the daily goals. This sample plan was written at 2,000 calories for a female Carb-Fueled Macro Type because, on average, this is approximately what my clients who fall into this category typically end up eating as a starting point. To scale this meal plan for a male Carb-Fueled Macro Type, multiply the portions by a factor of 1.6. Because we know the targeted percentages for protein, carbs, and fat, the macronutrients targeted were translated into grams by following the basic math in step #5 of determining your macronutrients (see page 146). In this sample meal plan, the target daily macronutrients are 215 grams carbs, 60 grams fat, and 150 grams protein.

MEAL PLAN FOR CARB-FUELED MACRO TYPE

Meal	Quantity	Food Description	Cal (kCal)	Carbs (g)	Fiber (g)	Fat (g)	Protein (g)
Pre-Workout	4 oz	Banana, raw	100.0	26.0	2.8	0.4	1.2
		Pre-Workout Total	**100.0**	**26.0**	**2.8**	**0.4**	**1.2**
Post-Workout	1 each	Strawberry-Pineapple Protein Shake (page 218)	177.0	12.0	1.0	3.0	25.0
		Post-Workout Total	**177.0**	**12.0**	**1.0**	**3.0**	**25.0**
Breakfast	1 serving	Breakfast Fried Rice (page 203)	309.0	30.0	2.0	7.0	31.0
		Breakfast Total	**309.0**	**30.0**	**2.0**	**7.0**	**31.0**
Snack	4 oz	Banana, raw	100.0	26.0	2.8	0.4	1.2
		Snack 1 Total	**100.0**	**26.0**	**2.8**	**0.4**	**1.2**
Lunch	6 oz (1½ servings)	Slow-Cooker Cilantro-Lime Chicken (page 206)	256.5	4.5	0.0	10.5	36.0
	10 oz (2½ servings)	Cumin-Cilantro Sweet Potatoes (page 252)	285.0	60.0	10.0	2.5	5.0

Meal	Quantity	Food Description	Cal (kCal)	Carbs (g)	Fiber (g)	Fat (g)	Protein (g)
	1 serving	Lemon-Garlic Kale Sauté (page 254)	36.0	7.0	1.0	0.0	2.0
		Lunch Total	**577.5**	**71.5**	**11.0**	**13.0**	**43.0**
Snack	1 each	Chocolate Chip Protein Blondies (page 239)	165.0	12.0	2.0	10.0	11.0
	2 oz	Banana, raw	50.0	13.0	1.4	0.2	0.6
		Snack 2 Total	**215**	**25.0**	**3.4**	**10.2**	**11.6**
Dinner	6 oz (1½ servings)	Slow-Cooker Cilantro-Lime Chicken (page 206)	256.5	4.5	0.0	10.5	36.0
	8 oz (2 servings)	Garlic-Jalapeño Cilantro Rice (page 247)	352.0	50.0	2.0	14.0	6.0
	1 each	Lemon-Garlic Kale Sauté (page 254)	36.0	7.0	1.0	0.0	2.0
		Dinner Total	**644.5**	**61.5**	**3.0**	**24.5**	**44.0**
			Cal (kCal)	Carbs (g)	Fiber (g)	Fat (g)	Protein (g)
		Your Daily Totals	2,123	**252**	26	**58.5**	**157**
		Your Daily Goal	2,000	**225**	17	**56**	**150**
		Target Macronutrient Percentages		**45%**		**25%**	**30%**

CARB-FUELED GROCERY LIST

	PROTEINS
☐	Whey Protein Isolate, Gauge Life Supplements
☐	Chicken breasts, boneless, skinless
☐	Egg whites
	CARBS
☐	Bananas, raw
☐	Strawberries, raw
☐	Pineapple, raw
☐	Almond extract
☐	Rice, long-grain white (Jasmine, Basmati)
☐	Sweet potatoes, raw (about 2 large)
☐	Peas, frozen
☐	Limes
☐	Garlic, raw
☐	Garlic powder
☐	Cayenne pepper
☐	Jalapeño
☐	Soy sauce (or coconut aminos)
☐	Sriracha hot sauce
☐	Chocolate chips
	FATS
☐	Olive oil
☐	Almond Butter, Justin's Classic
☐	Unsweetened almond milk
☐	Bacon

Type 2: Protein-Fueled Macro Type

SAMPLE 1,500-CALORIE MEAL PLAN

39% Protein | 32.5% Carbs | 28.5% Fats

Overview

Protein-fueled nutrition plans tend to be for those who gain and lose weight easily when they're focused (aka mesomorphs). These plans have a much higher amount of protein per meal, with a daily focus on getting *enough* protein. Most protein-fueled nutrition plans include a total caloric intake at least 500 calories lower than your TDEE. These plans range between 1,200 and 1,700 calories for most women and between 1,700 and 2,300 calories for most men. Remember, these values will vary based on the rate at which you want to pursue your goal. When eating according to a higher-protein protocol, especially for the first time, it's difficult to hit your macro ratios without a game plan. For this reason, I don't advise starting a protein-fueled protocol with flexible dieting (see page 194). I suggest following a meal plan for at least three weeks to get a feel for what portions and foods you need to eat.

Pre-Workout Nutrition

I advise getting at least 15 grams of carbs pre-workout if you're training first thing in the morning. If you work out later in the day, your last meal can serve as your pre-workout meal.

Post-Workout Nutrition

I advise consuming at least 25 grams of protein and at least 5 grams of carbs after working out. It's important to keep the fat content very low in your post-workout meal so as not to slow down your body's absorption of proteins to support muscle recovery and growth.[1] It's also important that you eat your post-workout meal within 30 to 45 minutes of training. Studies show that waiting 2 hours or longer to eat after a workout slows down glycogen synthesis by at least 50 percent.[2]

Meal Timing

High-protein nutrition is scientifically proven to boost your feeling of fullness.[3][4] If you are used to eating meals higher in carbs and fats, which are common in the standard American diet, the abrupt shift in your experience of fullness on this eating style will be a pleasant surprise. If you are used to eating larger portions of carbs, you can combine meals and eat two larger meals with high-protein snacks in between instead of three main meals. There is a common myth that the body can only absorb a maximum of 20 to 30 grams of protein per meal or snack, and it is therefore best to split your protein into five or six meals a day. This is false. The reality is the body has an unlimited ability to absorb amino acids.

Intermittent fasting is not necessary for those with a moderate carb tolerance. There is no issue, however, if you want to include it.

I suggest waiting 2 to 4 hours between meals with the exception of your post-workout meal. Once you have a post-workout shake, you are welcome to eat your next meal right away. For example, if you hit the gym in the early morning, you would eat a snack before the gym, then drink a post-workout shake within 30 minutes of working out. After that, you don't need to wait to eat breakfast or the next meal if you train later in the day.

Snacks

It is crucial that every snack you consume is protein-based. This presents a big shift if you are used to snacking on carbs. Read food labels to get a gauge for which snacks are highest in protein and which contain some protein but are dominant in other macronutrients. Granola, for instance, may seem like a healthy choice as it consists of natural ingredients like nuts and dried fruit. If you read the label, however, you'll see that it's high in carbs and fat, much lower in protein, and not the most suitable snack. You will need to choose foods high in protein and lower in carbs and fats. These include protein shakes and bars, almonds, nuts, seeds, string cheese, cottage cheese, Greek yogurt, beef jerky, deli meat, eggs, tuna, sardines, and more.

For those struggling to hit their protein intake, protein supplementation can be helpful. It is a convenient and economical way to hit your protein goals. There is nothing wrong with getting a substantial portion of your protein intake from supplements if that is easier for you. However, keep in mind that it is possible to hit your macros with real whole foods alone.

The Plan

The chart that follows outlines a sample meal plan broken down into a full day of eating for a Protein-Fueled Macro Type. The target daily caloric intake for this meal plan is 1,500 calories at 39 percent protein, 32.5 percent carbs, and 28.5 percent fat.

The menu is broken down into pre- and post-workout meals, breakfast, lunch, dinner, and snacks. It is written as though you are working out first thing in the morning. If you work out at a different time of day, simply move the pre- and post-workout meals accordingly.

Each meal is broken down into each food, quantity, and macronutrient per line. It is organized in this manner so you can see precisely how each food contributes to each meal, as well as the bigger picture of the entire day. This is particularly useful in making substitutions so you know exactly how much of each macronutrient you need to substitute. You will notice that every meal includes protein with the exception of the pre-workout meal. It is key to focus meals around protein while including moderate amounts of carbs and lower levels of dietary fats.

At the bottom of the chart, you will see the daily totals of calories, carbs, fiber, fat, and protein intake compared to the daily goals. This sample plan was written at 1,500 calories for a female Protein-Fueled Macro Type because, on average, this is approximately what my clients who fall into this category typically end up eating as a starting point. This value may be more or less based on your BMR and your activity level. To scale this meal plan for a male Carb-Fueled Macro Type, multiply the portions by a factor of 1.6. Because we know the targeted percentages for protein, carbs, and fat, the macronutrients targeted were translated into grams by following the basic math in step #5 of determining your macronutrients (see page 146). In this sample meal plan, the target daily macronutrients are 122 grams carbs, 48 grams fat, and 146 grams protein.

MEAL PLAN FOR PROTEIN-FUELED MACRO TYPE

Meal	Quantity	Food Description	Cal (kCal)	Carbs (g)	Fiber (g)	Fat (g)	Protein (g)
Pre-Workout	2 oz	Banana, raw	50.0	13.0	1.4	0.2	0.6
		Pre-Workout Total	**50.0**	**13.0**	**1.4**	**0.2**	**0.6**
Post-Workout	1 each	Antioxidant Detox Smoothie (page 215)	239.0	17.0	5.0	8.0	28.0
		Post-Workout Total	**239.0**	**17.0**	**5.0**	**8.0**	**28.0**
Breakfast	1 serving	Chicken Breakfast Sausage Fried Rice (page 204)	263.0	21.0	2.0	9.0	22.0
		Breakfast Total	**263.0**	**21.0**	**2.0**	**9.0**	**22.0**
Lunch	6 oz (1½ servings)	Filipino-Style Chicken Adobo (page 208)	270.0	7.5	0.0	13.5	28.5
	4 oz (1 serving)	Garlic-Jalapeño Cilantro Rice (page 247)	176.0	25.0	1.0	7.0	3.0
	1 serving	Lemon-Garlic Kale Sauté (page 254)	36.0	7.0	1.0	0.0	2.0
		Lunch Total	**482.0**	**39.5**	**2.0**	**20.5**	**33.5**
Snack	1 serving	Apple-Cinnamon Protein Pudding (page 241)	165.0	17.0	4.0	0.0	25.0
		Snack Total	**165.0**	**17.0**	**4.0**	**0.0**	**25.0**

Meal	Quantity	Food Description	Cal (kCal)	Carbs (g)	Fiber (g)	Fat (g)	Protein (g)
Dinner	6 oz (1½ servings)	Tequila-Lemon Flank Steak (page 205)	238.5	6.0	1.5	10.5	28.5
	1 serving	Asparagus Sauté (page 256)	69.0	5.0	4.0	4.0	6.0
		Dinner Total	**307.5**	**11.0**	**5.5**	**14.5**	**34.5**
			Cal (kCal)	Carbs (g)	Fiber (g)	Fat (g)	Protein (g)
		Your Daily Totals	1,506.5	**118.5**	19.9	**52.2**	**143.6**
		Your Daily Goal	1,500	**122**	17	**48**	**146**
		Macronutrient Percentages		**33%**		**28%**	**39%**

PROTEIN-FUELED GROCERY LIST

	PROTEINS
☐	Whey Protein Isolate, Gauge Life Supplements
☐	Chicken Maple Breakfast Sausage (Trader Joe's)
☐	Chicken thighs, boneless, skinless
☐	Flank steak
	CARBS
☐	Bananas, raw
☐	Blueberries, raw
☐	Apple slices, raw

☐	Apples, chopped, raw
☐	Kale
☐	Spinach
☐	Asparagus
☐	Rice, long-grain white
☐	Balsamic vinegar
☐	Garlic, raw
☐	Bay leaves
☐	Soy sauce (or coconut aminos)
☐	Lemons
☐	Jalapeño
☐	Cilantro, fresh, chopped
☐	Vanilla extract
☐	Xanthan gum
☐	Ground cinnamon
☐	Calorie-free sweetener packets (2g/each)
☐	Garlic powder
☐	Tequila
	FATS
☐	Olive oil
☐	Olive oil spray
☐	Kalamata olives, pitted
☐	Flaxseed
☐	Unsweetened coconut milk
☐	Bacon

Type 3: Protein-Fueled/Low-Carb Macro Type

SAMPLE 1,500-CALORIE MEAL PLAN

37.5% Protein| 26.5% Carbs | 36% Fats

Overview

Protein-fueled nutrition plans tend to be for those who gain and lose weight easily when they're focused (aka mesomorphs). However, an increasing number of individuals struggle with their carb tolerance. They need to bring their carb intake down but not so low that they're on a keto-style nutrition plan. This hybrid approach tends to be ideal for those over 35 who struggle with carb sensitivity or those in the beginning stages of prediabetes.

Protein-fueled/low-carb nutrition plans for people with a low carb tolerance need to be carefully dialed in for activity levels and tend to include a caloric deficit of at least 500 calories. Some, however, do better with a smaller caloric deficit and a slower rate of progress (between 0.5 and 1 pound of body fat lost per week). Taking too aggressive an approach to fat loss can work against those who have been overdieting for years. These plans range between 1,200 and 1,800 calories for most women and between 1,700 and 2,400 calories for most men. Remember that these values vary depending on the rate at which you wish to approach your goal.

For those with a low carb tolerance, eating according to a higher-protein protocol is a big adjustment for the first four to seven days, especially if it's your first time. In most cases, this is due to a natural sugar detox. You can expect to experience this if you have been eating more carbs than your body needs. If you have a thyroid issue, it is not advised to immediately jump into an aggressive caloric deficit. I advise that you begin at maintenance calories or at a slight deficit of ½ pound per week, only making modest adjustments and being cautious to not go above a deficit of 1 pound per week.

I don't advise starting this style of eating with flexible dieting (see page 194) alone. I suggest following a meal plan for a minimum of twenty-one days to get a feel for what portions and foods you need to eat. The biggest shift you will experience is in the type of carbs you need to eat. You may be use to starchy carbs like bread, rice, pasta, snacks, chips, and fries, and while you can still enjoy these in moderation, you will need to shift to carbs that are higher in fiber and lower on the glycemic index scale, meaning they do not cause a sharp spike in blood sugar. Foods such as root vegetables, leafy greens, cruciferous veggies, squash, and low-sugar fruit should become your new staples. You may find yourself trying new foods and experiencing a new sense of fullness from foods you never imagined eating, let alone enjoying. *Spaghetti squash? What?*

Pre-Workout Nutrition

I advise getting at least 10 grams of carbs pre-workout if you are training first thing in the morning. If you work out later in the day, your last meal can serve as your pre-workout meal.

Post-Workout Nutrition

I advise consuming at least 25 grams of protein and at least 5 grams of carbs after working out. It's important to keep the fat content very low in your post-workout meal so as not to slow down the body's absorption of proteins to support muscle recovery and growth.[5] While you can have a bit more fats than moderately carb-tolerant individuals, remember to keep these extra fats out of your post-workout meal. There is nothing wrong with including fats in a meal-replacement-style smoothie but not after a resistance workout.

Meal Timing

If you are just starting out, three main meals with pre- and post-work-out snacks are ideal. This is not the only way to approach this, but it tends to work the best for most. Those following this eating style also do well with intermittent fasting, as it minimizes insulin spikes by concentrating them in a shorter window. This doesn't mean eating less, but that you will do best concentrating your eating in an 8- to 12-hour window, where 8 hours are better than 12. This schedule often looks like a brunch-style meal and an early dinner, with snacks throughout the day to round out the macros.

Snacks

Snacks on this eating style tend to be fatty protein sources such as nuts, seeds, whole eggs, and cheese, although many on this plan don't eat any snacks at all. My clients who follow this eating style do best by eating slightly larger meals to boost satiety and using black coffee, hot tea, sparkling water, and countless foods (see page 152) as snacks. A *countless* food is an item so low in calories that you can include it in any meal without having to consider the added calories. These include foods like dill pickles, cucumbers, leafy greens, homemade kale chips, kimchi, sauerkraut, hot peppers, and green veggies.

The Plan

The chart that follows outlines a sample meal plan broken down into a full day of eating for a Protein-Fueled/Low-Carb Macro Type. The target daily caloric intake for this meal plan is 1,500 calories at 37.5 percent protein, 26.5 percent carbs, and 36 percent fat.

The menu is broken down into pre- and post-workout meals, breakfast, lunch, dinner, and snacks. It is written as though you are working out first thing in the morning. If you work out at a different time of day, simply move the pre- and post-workout meals accordingly.

Each meal is broken down into each food, quantity, and macronutrient per line. It is organized in this manner so you can see precisely how each food contributes to the meal, as well as the bigger picture of the entire day. This is particularly useful in making substitutions so you know exactly how much of each macronutrient you need to substitute. You will notice that every meal includes protein with the exception of the pre-workout meal. It is key to focus meals around fatty protein sources, going slightly lower in carbs.

At the bottom of the chart, you will see the daily totals of calories, carbs, fiber, fat, and protein intake compared to the daily goals. This sample plan was written at 1,500 calories for a female Protein-Fueled/Low-Carb Macro Type because, on average, this is approximately what my clients who fall into this category typically end up eating as a starting point. This value may be more or less, based on your BMR and your activity level. To scale this meal plan for a male Protein-Fueled/Low-Carb Macro Type, multiply the portions by a factor of 1.6. Because we know the targeted percentages for protein, carbs, and fat, the macronutrients targeted were translated into grams by following the basic math in step #5 of determining your macronutrients (see page 146). In this sample meal plan, the target daily macronutrients are 99 grams carbs, 60 grams fat, and 141 grams protein.

MEAL PLAN FOR PROTEIN-FUELED/
LOW-CARB MACRO TYPE

Meal	Quantity	Food Description	Cal (kCal)	Carbs (g)	Fiber (g)	Fat (g)	Protein (g)
Pre-Workout	2 oz	Banana, raw	50.0	13.0	1.4	0.2	0.6
		Pre-Workout Total	**50.0**	**13.0**	**1.4**	**0.2**	**0.6**
Post-Workout	1 each	Cantaloupe-Kale-Chia Protein Shake (page 213)	206.0	15.0	6.0	3.0	30.0
		Post-Workout Total	**206.0**	**15.0**	**6.0**	**3.0**	**30.0**
Breakfast	1 serving	Feta and Red Pepper Vegetarian Quiche (page 232)	255.0	4.0	1.0	20.0	15.0
		Breakfast Total	**255.0**	**4.0**	**1.0**	**20.0**	**15.0**
Lunch	6 oz (1½ servings)	Thai-Style Basil Chicken (page 212)	205.5	3.0	0.0	6.0	36.0
	4 oz (1 serving)	Garlic-Jalapeño Cilantro Rice (page 247)	176.0	25.0	1.0	7.0	3.0
	1 serving	Lemon-Garlic Kale Sauté (page 254)	36.0	7.0	1.0	0.0	2.0
		Lunch Total	**417.5**	**35.0**	**2.0**	**13.0**	**41.0**
Snack	1 each	Mixed Berry–Almond Protein Shake (page 214)	173.0	7.0	2.0	4.0	26.0
		Snack Total	**173.0**	**7.0**	**2.0**	**4.0**	**26.0**

Meal	Quantity	Food Description	Cal (kCal)	Carbs (g)	Fiber (g)	Fat (g)	Protein (g)
Dinner	1 serving	Salmon with Parmesan and Garlic-Rosemary Butter (page 224)	352.0	0.4	0.0	23.0	33.0
	4 oz	Rosemary-Roasted Butternut Squash (page 258)	55.0	13.0	3.0	0.0	1.0
		Dinner Total	**407.0**	**13.4**	**3.0**	**23.0**	**34.0**
			Cal (kCal)	Carbs (g)	Fiber (g)	Fat (g)	Protein (g)
		Your Daily Totals	1,508.5	**87.4**	15.4	**63.2**	**146.6**
		Your Daily Goal	1,500	**99**	17	**60**	**141**
		Macronutrient Percentages		**27%**		**36%**	**38%**

PROTEIN-FUELED/LOW-CARB GROCERY LIST

	PROTEINS
☐	Whey Protein Isolate, Gauge Life Supplements
☐	Whole eggs, large
☐	Chicken breasts, boneless, skinless
☐	Salmon fillet with skin
☐	Parmesan cheese, grated
	CARBS
☐	Bananas, raw
☐	Cantaloupe, cubed
☐	Mixed berries, frozen
☐	Red bell pepper, medium
☐	Kale
☐	Spinach

PROTEIN-FUELED / LOW-CARB GROCERY LIST *(cont.)*

☐	Jalapeño
☐	Rice, long-grain white
☐	Butternut squash
☐	Distilled white vinegar
☐	Garlic, raw
☐	Soy sauce (or coconut aminos)
☐	Lemon
☐	Bird's beak chile peppers, dried
☐	Cilantro, fresh, chopped
☐	Thai basil, fresh, chopped
☐	Rosemary, fresh
☐	Almond extract
☐	Black pepper, dried
☐	Thyme, dried
☐	Rosemary, dried
	FATS
☐	Olive oil
☐	Olive oil spray
☐	Salted grass-fed butter
☐	Heavy whipping cream
☐	Crumbled feta cheese
☐	Chia seeds
☐	Unsweetened almond milk

Type 4: Fat-Fueled Macro Type

SAMPLE 1,500-CALORIE MEAL PLAN
27.5% Protein | 17.5% Carbs | 55% Fats

Overview

Fat-fueled nutrition plans tend to be for those who gain weight easily and struggle to drop body fat (aka endomorphs). In most cases, this approach is ideal for those with hormonal imbalances, PCOS, prediabetes, a lower carb tolerance level, or who are trying to conceive. This plan is great for those who know they need to dial down the carbs but aren't willing to give them *all* up.

Fat-fueled nutrition plans for those with a low carb tolerance need to be carefully dialed in for activity levels and tend to include a caloric deficit of at least 500 calories. The journey will be slower for those in this boat than the first three macro types. If you have a hormonal imbalance, it is important to first approach your nutrition from a state of rebalancing your hormones for at least one to three weeks. This means eating at the suggested macro ratios but only calculated at your specific maintenance calories (aka your TDEE). It's important to take this step first because you most likely are experiencing nutrient deficiencies and need to allow your body some time to rebalance hormonally before approaching a caloric deficit. These plans range between 1,200 and 1,700 calories for most women and 1,700 and 2,300 calories for most men. Remember, these values will vary based on the rate at which you want to approach your goal. Eating according to a higher-fat, lower-carb protocol with a low carb tolerance, especially if it's your first time, is an adjustment for the first seven days. In most cases, this is due to a natural sugar detox your body will go through if you are used to eating many more carbs than your body needs.

I don't advise starting this style of eating with flexible dieting (see page 194) alone. I suggest following a meal plan for at least twenty-one days to get a feel for what portions and foods you need to eat. The biggest shift you will experience is in the *types* of carbs and proteins you should eat. You are probably used to starchy carbs like bread, rice, pasta, snacks, chips, and fries. This does not mean you can't have these foods anymore, but you need to monitor your portion size and frequency. Foods like winter and summer squash, root vegetables, leafy greens, cruciferous veggies, and low-sugar fruit will become your new staples. My most successful clients on this eating style are those who are the most open-minded to new ways of fueling their body.

Pre-Workout Nutrition

I advise getting at least 10 grams of carbs pre-workout if you are training first thing in the morning. If you work out later in the day, your last meal can serve as your pre-workout meal.

Post-Workout Nutrition

I advise consuming at least 25 grams of protein with at least 5 grams of carbs after working out. It's important to keep the fat content very low in your post-workout meal so as not to slow down the body's absorption of proteins to support muscle recovery and growth.[6] While you can have slightly higher fats than moderately carb tolerant individuals, remember to keep the extra fats out of your post-workout meal. There is nothing wrong with including fats in a meal-replacement-style smoothie, just not right after a resistance workout.

Meal Timing

If you are just starting out, three main meals with a pre- and post-workout snack are ideal. Although not the only way to approach this, it tends to work the best for most. This macro type also does well with intermittent fasting because it minimizes their insulin spikes throughout the day by concentrating them in a shorter window. This doesn't mean eating less but rather concentrating your eating within 8 to 12 hours, where 8 is better than 12. This often looks like a brunch-style meal and an early dinner, with snacks throughout the day and to round out the macros.

Snacks

Snacks on this eating style tend to look like fatty protein sources such as nuts, seeds, whole eggs, seeds, and cheese, if you have any snacks at all. My clients who follow this eating style do best by eating larger meals to boost satiety and using black coffee, hot tea, sparkling water, and *countless* foods (see page 152) as snacks.

The Plan

The chart that follows outlines a sample meal plan broken down into a full day of eating for a Fat-Fueled Macro Type. The target daily caloric intake for this meal plan is 1,500 calories at 27.5 percent protein, 17.5 percent carbs, and 55 percent fat.

The menu is broken down into pre- and post-workout meals, breakfast, lunch, dinner, and snacks. It is written as though you are working out first thing in the morning. If you work out at a different time of day, simply move the pre- and post-workout meals accordingly.

Each meal is broken down into each food, quantity, and macronutrient per line. It is organized in this manner so you can see precisely how each food contributes to the meal, as well as the bigger picture of the entire day. This is particularly useful in making substitutions so you know exactly how much of each macronutrient you need to substitute. You will notice that the meals tend to be higher in fatty proteins and moderate in high-fiber carbs like veggies cooked with healthy fats like olive oil, while being lower in starchy carbs.

At the bottom of the chart, you will see the daily totals of calories, carbs, fiber, fat, and protein intake compared to the daily goals. This sample plan was written at 1,500 calories for a female Fat-Fueled Macro Type because, on average, this is approximately what my clients who fall into this category typically end up eating as a starting point. To scale this meal plan for a male Fat-Fueled Macro Type, multiply the portions by a factor of 1.6. Because we know the targeted percentages for protein, carbs, and fat, the macronutrients targeted were translated into grams by following the basic math in step #5 of determining your macronutrients (see page 146). In this sample meal plan, the target daily macronutrients are 66 grams carbs, 92 grams fat, and 103 grams protein.

MEAL PLAN FOR FAT-FUELED MACRO TYPE

Meal	Quantity	Food Description	Cal (kCal)	Carbs (g)	Fiber (g)	Fat (g)	Protein (g)
Pre-Workout	3 oz	Apple, raw	45.0	12.0	2.1	0.0	0.0
		Pre-Workout Total	**45.0**	**12.0**	**2.1**	**0.0**	**0.0**
Post-Workout	1 each	Mixed Berry–Almond Protein Shake (page 214)	173.0	7.0	2.0	4.0	26.0
		Post-Workout Total	**173.0**	**7.0**	**2.0**	**4.0**	**26.0**
Breakfast	1 serving	Feta and Red Pepper Vegetarian Quiche (page 232)	255.0	4.0	1.0	20.0	15.0
	3 oz	Avocado	135.0	7.2	5.7	12.6	2.1
		Breakfast Total	**390.0**	**11.2**	**6.7**	**32.6**	**17.1**
Lunch	1 serving	Salmon with Parmesan and Garlic-Rosemary Butter (page 224)	352.0	0.4	0.0	23.0	33.0
	1 serving	Lemon-Garlic Kale Sauté (page 254)	36.0	7.0	1.0	0.0	2.0

Meal	Quantity	Food Description	Cal (kCal)	Carbs (g)	Fiber (g)	Fat (g)	Protein (g)
	3 oz (¾ serving)	Oven-Roasted Spiced Potatoes (page 250)	128.3	21.0	3.0	5.3	3.0
		Lunch Total	**516.3**	**28.4**	**4.0**	**28.3**	**38.0**
Dinner	3 slices	Garlic and Mushroom White Pizza (page 225)	408	6.0	1.2	30	27.0
		Dinner Total	**408**	**6.0**	**1.2**	**30**	**27.0**
			Cal (kCal)	Carbs (g)	Fiber (g)	Fat (g)	Protein (g)
		Your Daily Totals	1,532	**64.6**	16	**94.9**	**108.1**
		Your Daily Goal	1,500	**66**	17	**92**	**103**
		Macronutrient Percentages		**17%**		**55%**	**28%**

FAT-FUELED GROCERY LIST

	PROTEINS
☐	Whey Protein Isolate, Gauge Life Supplements
☐	Whole eggs, large
☐	Full-fat mozzarella cheese, shredded
☐	Salmon fillet with skin
☐	Parmesan cheese, grated
	CARBS
☐	Apple slices
☐	Mixed berries, frozen
☐	Red bell pepper, medium
☐	Kale
☐	Spinach

FAT-FUELED GROCERY LIST *(cont.)*

☐	Cauliflower rice, frozen
☐	Mushrooms
☐	Garlic, raw
☐	Lemon
☐	Basil, fresh
☐	Rosemary, fresh
☐	Almond extract
☐	Black pepper, dried
☐	Thyme, dried
☐	Rosemary, dried
	FATS
☐	Olive oil
☐	Olive oil spray
☐	Salted grass-fed butter
☐	Heavy whipping cream
☐	Crumbled feta cheese
☐	Avocado
☐	Unsweetened almond milk

Type 5: Fat-Fueled/Low-Carb Macro Type

SAMPLE 1,500-CALORIE MEAL PLAN
20% Protein | 5% Carbs | 75% Fat

Overview

Fat-Fueled/Low-Carb Macro types benefit from a ketogenic diet. In most cases, this eating style is for those who tend to easily gain weight but struggle to drop body fat (aka endomorphs). However, those with other body types can also thrive on this approach. Keto is ideal for you if you are ready for a nutritional overhaul and are sick of feeling tired, lethargic, and bloated. It's not that you don't like or enjoy carbs, but you don't like how they make you feel. Carbs give you brain fog, your weight loss is at a complete standstill, and your energy is nonexistent. This approach is great for those with hormonal imbalances, PCOS, prediabetes, diabetes, or an extremely low carb tolerance.

Fat-fueled/low-carb nutrition plans need to be carefully dialed in for activity levels and tend to include a caloric deficit of at least 500 calories. These plans tend to range between 1,200 and 1,700 calories for most women and 1,700 and 2,300 calories for most men. Remember, these values will vary based on the rate at which you wish to approach your goal. Eating according to a keto protocol for the first time is an adjustment for the first four to seven days. Many people experience what is known as the keto flu when first starting a keto plan, which is an electrolyte imbalance that can make you feel nauseated and light-headed for one to three days. When you drop your carb intake, your body shifts from using carbs for fuel to fat, and your insulin levels drop (this is the whole idea of going keto). However, insulin sends messages to the kidneys to retain a certain amount of sodium, potassium, and magnesium, so when insulin is low, the kidneys will expel much higher levels of these electrolytes, leading to the lightheaded and dizzy feeling. You can address this by increasing your salt intake, up to five times the RDA of sodium for the day since your body is expelling and not retaining it.

I do not advise starting this style of eating with flexible dieting (see page 194) alone. I suggest following a meal plan for at least twenty-one days to get a feel for what portions and foods you need to eat. The biggest shift you will experience is in the *type* of carbs you can eat, which now only includes low-sugar fruit, veggies, and leafy greens. You may also find hitting your fat intake much harder than you imagined. You will be able to eat steak, butter, avocado, nuts, salmon, cheese, and a variety of other high-fat foods that you may have considered off-limits in the past.

Pre-Workout Nutrition

I advise getting at least 10 grams of fat prior to working out; however, you are welcome to skip a pre-workout snack on keto. Your body will be relying on fat for fuel, and when you are in ketosis, your body can pull from stored body fat for fuel.

Post-Workout Nutrition

On keto, post-workout nutrition is only crucial if you are weight training at an intense level. If you are doing light cardio, a special post-workout meal isn't necessary. You are welcome to make your next natural meal your post-workout meal.

If you do eat a post-workout meal, I advise consuming 10 grams of protein with at least 5 grams of carbs. It's important to keep the fat content very low in your post-workout meal so as not to slow down the body's absorption of proteins, to support muscle recovery and growth.[7] Keeping the fat content lower in post-workout meals is ideal for a ketogenic diet, as fat slows the body's digestion of protein.

Meal Timing

Those following this eating style also do well with intermittent fasting, because it minimizes their insulin spikes throughout the day by concentrating them in a shorter window. For example, having a coffee with a healthy fat in the morning, waiting until 11 a.m. to 12 p.m. for their first meal, and ending their eating window by 7 to 8 p.m. works best for most.

Snacks

Snacks on this eating style tend to look like fatty protein sources such as nuts, seeds, whole eggs, and cheese. It is not necessary to include snacks, as you will feel very full from the high fat content. Most people feel so full that not only do cravings disappear, but they find it hard to eat because their level of satiety is so high. It's important to eliminate carb-based snacks and only seek out foods that enable you to remain in a state of nutritional ketosis.

The Plan

The chart that follows outlines a sample meal plan broken down into a full day of eating for a Fat-Fueled/Low-Carb Macro Type (aka the ketogenic diet). The target daily caloric intake for this meal plan is 1,500 calories at 20 percent protein, 5 percent carbs, and 75 percent fat.

The menu is broken down into pre- and post-workout meals, breakfast, lunch, dinner, and snacks. It is written as though you are working out first thing in the morning. If you work out at a different time of day, simply move the pre- and post-workout meals accordingly.

Each meal is broken down into each food, quantity, and macronutrient per line. It is organized in this manner so you can see precisely how each food contributes to the meal, as well as the bigger picture of the entire day. This is particularly useful in making substitutions so you know exactly how much of each macronutrient you need to substitute. You will notice that the meals tend to be higher in fatty proteins, moderate in high-fiber carbs such as veggies cooked with healthy fats like olive oil, while being significantly lower in starchy carbs.

At the bottom of the chart, you will see the daily totals of calories, carbs, fiber, fat, and protein intake compared to the daily goals. This sample plan was written at 1,500 calories for a female Fat-Fueled/Low-Carb Macro Type because, on average, this is approximately what my clients who fall into this category typically end up eating as a starting point. To scale this meal plan for a male Fat-Fueled/Low-Carb Macro

Type, multiply the portions by a factor of 1.6. Because we know the targeted percentages for protein, carbs, and fat, the macronutrients targeted were translated into grams by following the basic math in step #5 of determining your macronutrients (see page 146). In this sample meal plan, the target daily macronutrients are 19 grams carbs, 117 grams fat, and 93 grams protein.

MEAL PLAN FOR FAT-FUELED/LOW-CARB MACRO TYPE

Meal	Quantity	Food Description	Cal (kCal)	Carbs (g)	Fiber (g)	Fat (g)	Protein (g)
Pre-Workout	8 oz	Coffee (regular or decaf)	0.0	0.0	0.0	0.0	0.0
	1 oz	Coconut butter (manna)	200.0	6.0	4.0	18.0	2.0
		Pre-Workout Total	**200.0**	**6.0**	**4.0**	**18.0**	**2.0**
Post-Workout	0.3 oz	Collagen Peptides, Unflavored, Prime, Gauge Life (1 scoop = 22 g/0.786 oz)	34.4	0.0	0.0	0.0	7.6
	8 oz	Almond milk, unsweetened	30.0	1.0	1.0	2.5	1.0
	1 oz	Strawberries, raw	9.0	2.2	0.6	0.1	0.2
		Post-Workout Total	**73.4**	**3.2**	**1.6**	**2.6**	**8.8**
Breakfast	4 oz	Eggs, large (1 egg = 2 oz)	143.0	1.0	0.0	10.0	13.0

Meal	Quantity	Food Description	Cal (kCal)	Carbs (g)	Fiber (g)	Fat (g)	Protein (g)
	0.5 oz	Bacon, Sunday, Applegate Naturals/ Organics (2 fried slices = 14 g/0.5 oz)	70.0	0.0	0.0	5.0	6.0
	1 serving	Lemon Garlic Kale Sauté (page 254)	36.0	7.0	1.0	0.0	2.0
		Breakfast Total	**249.0**	**8.0**	**1.0**	**15.0**	**21.0**
Lunch	1 serving	Salmon with Parmesan and Garlic-Rosemary Butter (page 224)	352.0	0.4	0.0	23.0	33.0
	1 serving	Lemon Garlic Kale Sauté (page 254)	36.0	7.0	1.0	0.0	2.0
	0.25 oz	Olive oil (1 Tbsp = 15 g/0.54 oz)	56.0	0.0	0.0	6.5	0.0
		Lunch Total	**444.0**	**7.4**	**1.0**	**29.5**	**35.0**
Snack	8 oz	Hot green tea	0.0	0.0	0.0	0.0	0.0
	2 servings	Hummus Deviled Eggs (page 225)	152.0	4.0	2.0	12.0	10.0
		Snack Total	**152.0**	**4.0**	**2.0**	**12.0**	**10.0**
Dinner	1 serving	Chimichurri Chicken Thighs (page 219)	308.0	4.0	1.0	23.0	20.0
	2 oz	Avocado	90.0	4.8	3.8	8.4	1.2
	1 oz	Spinach, raw	7.0	1.0	1.0	0.0	1.0
	0.25 oz	Olive oil (1 Tbsp = 15 g/0.54 oz)	56.0	0.0	0.0	6.5	0.0
		Dinner Total	**461.0**	**9.8**	**5.8**	**37.9**	**22.2**

		Cal (kCal)	Carbs (g)	Fiber (g)	Fat (g)	Protein (g)
	Your Daily Totals	1,579.4	**38.4**	15.4	**115**	**99**
	Your Daily Goal	1,500	**19**	17	**117**	**93**
	Macronutrient Percentages		5%		75%	20%

FAT-FUELED/LOW-CARB GROCERY LIST

	PROTEINS
☐	Collagen Peptides, Gauge Life Supplements
☐	Whole eggs, large
☐	Salmon fillet with skin
☐	Parmesan cheese, grated
☐	Chicken thighs, bone-in
	CARBS
☐	Strawberries
☐	Mixed berries, frozen
☐	Red bell pepper, medium
☐	Kale
☐	Spinach
☐	Garlic, raw
☐	Lemon
☐	Limes
☐	Cilantro, fresh, chopped
☐	Italian parsley, fresh, chopped
☐	Rosemary, fresh
☐	Jalapeño
☐	Cumin, ground
☐	Oregano, dried

	FATS
☐	Olive oil
☐	Olive oil spray
☐	Coconut butter (manna)
☐	Bacon
☐	Salted grass-fed butter
☐	Hummus
☐	Avocado
☐	Unsweetened almond milk
	MISCELLANEOUS
☐	Green tea
☐	Coffee

8

Cooking for Your Macro Type

Now that we know the science behind nutrition and macros, it's time to apply what we've learned to the kitchen! Lack of planning is the number one reason people fall off track with their nutrition. The difference between reaching your goals by staying on track and falling victim to the inconveniences of everyday life is planning your meals to fit your macros.

If you have never cooked in bulk, meal planning can seem overwhelming, but I promise, it's simple to master. Not only does it make you more organized, but it also saves you time and money. When you meal prep, you arrange your foods and recipes like the pieces of a puzzle, where the overall picture is your daily protein, carb, and fat content.

Although a detailed macro-based meal plan makes it easy to stay on track, it's not always practical for those with busy lifestyles. If this is you, a flexible dieting approach will also work. **Flexible dieting** means using a macro-tracking app that enables you to look up foods in an online database as you eat them and record the amount you consumed. This will automatically calculate the amounts of protein, carbs, and fats you consume in a day relative to your daily targets, making it easy for you to freely choose foods as long as you stay within your macronutrient goals for the day. The reason this method is so appealing is because absolutely nothing is off limits. This means you can actually have unconventional "diet" foods like pizza as long as you track the food and adjust your food intake for the balance of the day to remain within your daily macro-nutrient targets for proteins, carbs, and fats. In order to drop body fat, it's not absolutely necessary to consume rigid, monotonous meals with little to no variety. As long as the sum of all the food you consume in a day fits your macros, you are good to go! This method is also commonly referred to as IIFYM or "if it fits your macros."

It takes some practice to get the hang of this approach. If you try this with no idea about macros, you will most likely go over certain macros and be under on others, so I recommend investing the time and energy in meal prep before using flexible dieting, if you can. Once you have some hands-on experience weighing and portioning your meals, you'll have a feel for what the correct portions look like for the foods you eat most often. Meal prepping also gives you a better foundation in budgeting your macros throughout the day to reach your goals.

First Steps

Before you meal prep, make sure to stock up on essential tools and spices. Having the correct items on hand is essential to making a successful transition to a healthy lifestyle. Equipping your kitchen and pantry with the proper materials makes it fun and easy to adopt healthier habits. Here are the tools that you'll need:

- Food scale
- Nontoxic nonstick skillet
- Cooking oil atomizer
- Nonstick baking sheet
- Parchment paper
- Measuring cups
- Measuring spoons
- Storage containers
- Supplements (optional)

Once you have the right equipment, the next step is to procure quality seasonings and spices. Flavor is a top priority! Do not be afraid to season your food! Always have a wide array of staple seasonings on hand to make even the simplest foods fun and flavorful. The following items offer a great starting point to create a wide variety of flavor profiles:

- Bay leaves
- Black pepper
- Cayenne pepper
- Chili powder
- Cinnamon, ground
- Coriander
- Cumin, ground
- Curry powder
- Garlic powder
- Ginger
- Oregano, dried
- Paprika
- Red pepper, crushed
- Rosemary, dried
- Sea salt, Himalayan (Note that I use Himalayan sea salt for all recipes.)
- Thyme, dried
- Turmeric

Now that you have the essentials, it's time to get down to business! Follow these three simple steps for pitch-perfect meal prep.

1. Organize Your Cooking Strategy

In preparing to follow your meal plan, you'll first want to determine the items you need to cook in advance. You may prefer to prepare a fresh breakfast every morning, or you may want something ready-made that you can eat on your commute to work. Once you know which meals to prepare in advance, you'll know where to focus your efforts. For example, if you like to cook breakfast most every morning, that leaves you with lunch, dinner, and snacks to prepare in advance. You won't have to cook most snacks, so it really boils down to preparing lunch and dinner.

Once you define your cooking strategy, you will need to consider your cooking methods. This means being mindful of ingredients that can add hidden calories to your daily meals without your realizing it. This includes condiments, dressings, cooking oils, alcohol, and beverages (i.e., sports drinks, soda, juice).

2. Identify What You Need to Cook Ahead of Time

Write or print out a copy of your meal plan, and circle which items you'll need to cook in advance. For example, if your lunches and dinners both have grilled chicken in them, you'll need to prepare a bunch of chicken in advance. If you have rice or sweet potatoes in more than one meal, prepare some in bulk to accommodate this. The more meals you can find that use food you prepare in bulk, the simpler your meal preparation will be.

3. Stage Your Ingredients

Whether you decide to cook for an entire week at once or to cook every meal from scratch, staging your ingredients is a *huge* key to success. *Staging* ingredients means prewashing and chopping your veggies so they are set and ready to go. It means portioning out the ingredients for your smoothies so all you need to do is dump a baggie into the blender. It means cooking your proteins in large batches and having them ready in a storage container for easy access when it's time to put a meal together. Any steps you can take to organize your ingredients in advance will make sticking to your plan ten times easier.

Cook for Your Macro Type

Now that you are ready to food prep, it's important to have fun recipes to prepare. This is the part where you can enjoy being creative with your meals. Living a healthy lifestyle with an eating plan for your body type can taste incredible! What follows are simple, delicious recipes that make this approach *practical*. If you want intricate, gourmet, bougie recipes, this is not the book for you. But if you want things that taste good, are easy to cook, won't break the bank, *and* that your family will enjoy, you are in the right place!

My cooking philosophy is all about preparing quality ingredients in a way that lets their natural flavors shine through. The true test of macro-based cooking is finding creative ways to explore flavor without adding chemical additives or cheap ingredients that artificially boost it — like refined sugars, hydrogenated oils, and flavorings full of salt-based preservatives. This takes some adjusting to. I encourage you to embrace it. You are transforming your body from the inside out, one molecule and cell at a time, as a direct result of the food you consume. Having the right recipes in your arsenal can be the key between hoping for improved health and taking the steps to accomplish it.

Many people fail at healthy living because they do not know how to cook. *Anyone* can make food tasty by adding an unlimited amount of sugar, fat, and salt. The real challenge is preparing foods with incredible flavor and macronutrients as a constraint. Whether you are terrified of the stove or are an experienced chef, you'll need to rethink everything you know about cooking.

Before you begin, drop all preconceived notions of what you think healthy food tastes like. The biggest misconception about healthy eating is that you need to sacrifice flavor and overall satisfaction. You may be mentally preparing yourself to "diet," getting ready to sacrifice delicious food in exchange for the body you've always wanted. If this is you, *stop*.

Macro-based cooking has a learning curve, but for the most part, you can become an expert macro-chef by following instructions. If you can boil a pot of water, you can cook delicious macro-friendly meals. Be patient with yourself, use the correct tools, and read the recipes all the way through. These recipes may include steps that are new to you, so read through each preparation step, and refrain from making assumptions.

Here are four overarching things to keep in mind to set you up for success when cooking in your macro-based kitchen:

BE CAREFUL ABOUT OVERCOOKING. The main mistake people make in macro-based cooking is applying too much heat to meats and veggies. When cooking lean meats, you have to pay more attention to managing moisture. Cooking low and slow, not overcooking, and using water, steam, broth, lemon, lime, or light marinades to infuse foods with flavor is key.

WATCH YOUR COOKING OILS. The oil you cook with counts toward your macros! This means avoiding heavy frying or sautéing with a lot of oil and getting used to sautéing in quality nonstick cooking pans. It also means grilling, broiling, baking on parchment paper, steaming, and air frying. You will need to be more mindful of the texture and moisture content of your food and how each method of preparation impacts that. This is more challenging with leaner meats. Don't worry about the effect of cooking with less oil though; this chapter is loaded with quality recipes that are juicy and delicious!

SUBSTITUTE WITH CAUTION. You can customize any of the recipes in this chapter to be more attuned to your palate. The key is to make sure your substitutions don't throw off your macros. If, for example, you are making the Thai-Style Basil Chicken (page 212) and decide to make the recipe with shrimp, your macros will remain on track because shrimp and chicken breast contain very similar amounts of protein and fat. However, if you swap chicken out for a fattier protein source like beef, you'll need to account for those extra calories.

RETHINK REHEATING. When cooking these recipes, consider leftovers and which items will and will not reheat well. Not everything you prepare can freeze and thaw without changing its flavor and texture. Before you cook any of these recipes in bulk, try them out and gain familiarity with them. Most proteins and starchy carbs reheat well, but veggies do not, so I recommend cooking veggies fresh each day if you are able to. But if you don't have time to go through the entire cooking process, you can still prep veggies in advance by washing, chopping, and staging them so they are ready to go.

A MIX-AND-MATCH APPROACH

The recipes in this chapter are arranged to correspond easily with the meal plan guidelines from Chapters 6 and 7. You'll find the recipes organized by category: Lean Proteins, Fatty Proteins, Fatty Low-GI Carbs, Protein Snacks, High-GI Carbs, Low-GI Carbs, and Healthy Fats. For example, if the guidelines for your macro type (page 155–159) suggest fatty proteins + low-GI carbs for a meal, you can look through the recipes in each respective category (in this case, choose a fatty protein and choose a low-GI carb) to find the ones that fit your palate.

Menu Template Category Examples

Fatty Protein		Lean Protein	
Eggs	Nut butter	Chicken breast	Branzino
Salmon	Cheese	Egg whites	Turkey breast
Duck	Beef burger	Shrimp	Lobster
Lamb	Chicken thighs	Sea bass	Trout
Rib eye	Chicken wings	Mahi mahi	Crab
Wagyu	Pork	Whey isolate	Snapper
Nuts	Bacon	Tenderloin	Scallops

Low-GI Carbs		High-GI Carbs	
Leafy greens	Tomato	Sweet potato	Grapes
Carrots	Legumes	Rice	Tortillas
Zucchini	Squash	Pasta	Pretzels
Broccoli	Blueberries	Sprouted bread	Dried fruit
Cauliflower	Peas	Oats	Plantains
Apples	String beans	Quinoa	Pineapple
Strawberries	Mushrooms	Banana	Corn
Peaches	Eggplant	Couscous	Mango

Menu Template Category Examples *(cont.)*

Fatty Low-GI Carbs	Healthy Fats	
Low-carb bread	Olive oil	Coconut oil
Almond flour tortillas	Pesto	Sesame oil
Coconut flour tortillas	Nuts	Chia seeds
Veggies sautéed in healthy fats	Seeds	Flax
Veggie casseroles	Avocado	Pumpkin seeds
Coconut chips	Avocado oil	Olives
Healthy sauces/dips (i.e., hummus)	Grass-fed butter	Walnuts
Nuts/nut butter + low-sugar fruit	Ghee	Almonds

I've handcrafted this simple collection of recipes with love and care, from my kitchen to yours. It can be challenging to become adept at making recipes that are delicious and healthy at the same time, but I've done that work for you! Many of my clients, family members, and friends tell me they do not feel like they are on a diet when they are using my recipes. This is one of the nicest compliments to receive. The following recipes are easy, simple, affordable, and family-friendly. Not only will they nourish you and your loved ones, but they will support your body transformation for years to come!

Lean Protein Recipes

Breakfast Fried Rice

Makes 1 serving
Prep Time: 5 minutes
Cook Time: 5 minutes

MEAL PLAN KEY: LEAN PROTEIN + HIGH-GI CARB

Welcome to my world of rice and bacon for breakfast with this savory yet effortless high-protein meal. This meal is family-friendly, budget-friendly, and makes meal prep something you actually look forward to. It can be enjoyed for breakfast, lunch, or dinner. Did I mention bacon? Yes, you can actually eat bacon every day and still drop body fat. I use organic peas, but you can use conventional.

Ingredients
    2 slices bacon
    2 cloves garlic, chopped
    6 oz (¾ cup) liquid egg whites (from about 6 large eggs)
    2 oz (¼ cup) frozen peas
    4 oz (½ cup) cooked white rice
    2 tablespoons soy sauce*
    ¼ teaspoon paprika
    Hot sauce (optional)
    Use coconut aminos for a soy-free alternative.

1. Panfry the bacon in a nonstick skillet using a nonmetal spatula until crisp. Transfer the bacon to a plate and set aside.
2. Add the garlic to the bacon grease in the pan and sauté over medium-high heat for 30 seconds, then reduce the heat to medium. Pour the egg whites into the skillet and scramble for 10 seconds. Add the peas and cover with lid for 30 seconds. Uncover and scramble the contents together for 15 seconds, or until the peas are bright green and no longer frozen.

3. Add the rice to the skillet and top with the soy sauce and paprika. Stir-fry together until all ingredients are equally distributed. Crumble the bacon and stir into the fried rice if you like, or simply serve as whole pieces on the side. Serve with hot sauce.

Meal Prep Tips
- If doubling or tripling recipe, allow the contents to cool at room temperature for 10 minutes before refrigerating.
- Keeps for 4 to 5 days refrigerated.
- Easy to prepare in bulk for 3 or more days at a time.

Macros per serving:
Calories (kCal) 309; Total Fat 7g (Saturated Fat 3g, Trans Fat 0g); Cholesterol 15mg; Sodium 1,123mg; Potassium 383mg; Total Carbohydrate 30g (Dietary Fiber 2g, Sugars 3g); Protein 31g

Chicken Breakfast Sausage Fried Rice

Makes 1 serving
Prep Time: 5 minutes
Cook Time: 5 minutes
MEAL PLAN KEY: LEAN PROTEIN + HIGH-GI CARB

I am a huge fan of the savory breakfast, especially when it's a recipe that can also be lunch or dinner! Cutting the sausage into slices allows for more surface area to crisp up and burn a little on the edge. I personally enjoy meats with that "almost burnt" flavor for added complexity in a meal, and this simple breakfast is no exception. I prefer to use organic rice.

Ingredients
Olive oil spray
1 clove garlic, minced
4 oz (4 links) Trader Joe's Chicken Maple Breakfast Sausage, cut into slices
1 oz (1 cup) spinach
4 oz (½ cup) cooked brown rice

Optional toppings: sriracha, scallions, jalapeños, onions, cilantro, or
   crushed red pepper

1. Lightly coat a nonstick skillet with a spray of olive oil and heat over
   medium-high heat. Add the garlic and sauté for 30 to 60 seconds. Add the
   sausage and cook over high heat, stirring, for 3 to 4 minutes, until lightly
   burnt.
2. Tightly ball the spinach on a cutting board and dice. Add the spinach to
   the skillet and stir-fry briefly with the sausage, then add 1 tablespoon of
   water and cover to steam the stir-fry for 30 seconds.
3. Add the rice to the skillet and stir until all ingredients are equally distributed, then remove from heat and plate. Serve immediately with your
   toppings of choice.

Meal Prep Tips
   • If doubling or tripling this recipe, allow to cool at room temperature for
     10 minutes before refrigerating.
   • Keeps for 4 to 5 days refrigerated.
   • Easy to prepare in bulk for 3 or more meals.

Macros per serving:
   Calories (kCal) 263; Total Fat 9g (Saturated Fat 3g, Trans Fat 0g); Cholesterol 59mg;
   Sodium 592mg; Potassium 179mg; Total Carbohydrate 21g (Dietary Fiber 2g, Sugars 0g);
   Protein 22g

Tequila-Lemon Flank Steak

Makes 8 servings
Prep Time: 5 minutes, plus 30 minutes marinating (or up to 24 hours)
Cook Time: 10 minutes
MEAL PLAN KEY: LEAN PROTEIN

Flank steak gets a surprising boost of flavor from tequila. Experience a
rich, juicy, and delicious macro-friendly meal that keeps your food far from
boring. This recipe is a perfect example of how macro-based cooking is all

about naturally enhancing flavor. Instead of dousing meats in low-quality processed seasonings, tequila, lemon, and garlic make for a well-balanced and well-seasoned dish. Enjoy as the meat for tacos or with a side of complex carbs or the veggies of your choice!

Ingredients

2 oz lemon juice (juice of ~2 lemons)

1 oz (2 tablespoons) tequila

2 oz (¼ cup) garlic powder

1 teaspoon sea salt

¼ teaspoon freshly ground black pepper

24 oz (1½ lb) flank steak

Fresh cilantro for garnish (optional)

1. In a small bowl, mix together the lemon juice, tequila, garlic powder, salt, and pepper and transfer to a gallon-size plastic bag. Shake the ingredients until well combined. Add the flank steak, seal, and rub the marinade into the meat until well covered. Marinate in the fridge for at least 30 minutes or up to 24 hours.
2. Remove the steak from the bag and let excess marinade drip off. Place the steak on the grill over medium-high heat (~350°F) and cook for about 6 minutes per side or to the temperature of your choice.
3. Transfer the steak to a cutting board and let rest for 5 minutes. Slice into thin slices, garnish with cilantro, and serve.

Macros per 4-ounce serving:

Calories (kCal) 159; Total Fat 7g (Saturated Fat 3g, Trans Fat 0g); Cholesterol 56mg; Sodium 357mg; Potassium 77mg; Total Carbohydrate 4g (Dietary Fiber 1g, Sugars 1g); Protein 19g

Slow-Cooker Cilantro-Lime Chicken

Makes 12 servings

Prep Time: 5 minutes

Cook Time: 4 to 6 hours

MEAL PLAN KEY: LEAN PROTEIN

I love shredded chicken, and this version is packed with flavor and absolutely delicious! Tender and juicy seasoned chicken breasts cook in the slow cooker with a flavorful and light cilantro lime sauce. Serve as a filling in tacos or burritos, over rice, on toast, or with the starchy carbs and veggies of your choice. I will often make large batches and freeze in meal-size portions.

Ingredients

48 oz (3 lb) boneless skinless chicken breasts

2 oz (¼ cup) extra-virgin olive oil

0.14 oz (¼ cup) chopped fresh cilantro

2 oz (¼ cup) water

2 oz (¼ cup) sriracha

3 cloves garlic, chopped

3 oz lime juice (juice of 3 limes squeezed)

Additional fresh cilantro and sriracha, for garnish (optional)

1. Combine all the ingredients in a slow cooker. Cover, set to low, and cook for 4 to 6 hours. (You'll need the full 6 hours if starting with frozen chicken.)
2. Once cooked, shred the chicken with two forks inside of the slow cooker; it should easily shred with little handling.
3. Serve immediately, topping with additional fresh cilantro and sriracha as desired.

Meal Prep Tips

- The shredded chicken is an easy make-ahead freezer meal. Or you can freeze it before cooking by tossing all the ingredients in a 1-gallon freezer plastic bag and popping it into the freezer. Thaw in the refrigerator the night before, then dump the ingredients in your slow cooker when you are ready to rock & roll!
- Easy to prepare in bulk for 3 or more meals.

Macros per serving:

Calories (kCal) 171; Total Fat 7g (Saturated Fat 2g, Trans Fat 0g); Cholesterol 56mg; Sodium 123mg; Potassium: 271mg; Total Carbohydrate 3g (Dietary Fiber 0g, Sugars 1g); Protein 24g

Filipino-Style Chicken Adobo

6 servings

Prep Time: 10 minutes

Cook Time: 45 minutes

MEAL PLAN KEY: LEAN PROTEIN

You'll get intense flavor depth from simple ingredients with this amazing yet healthy Filipino-inspired chicken. When I was growing up, adobo was always the ultimate crowd pleaser at every potluck. The original is so high in fat that it could be enjoyed only occasionally, but this lighter version can be a part of your weekly meal rotation. The chicken is great for serving at a family dinner, potluck, or holiday gathering and pairs well with white or brown rice, string beans, asparagus, spinach, or the veggie of your choice.

Ingredients

32 oz (4 cups) water

24 oz (1½ lb) boneless skinless chicken thighs or skinless drumsticks (recipe also works well with pork belly or pork shoulder)

4 oz (½ cup) soy sauce*

4 oz (½ cup) balsamic vinegar

6 cloves garlic, chopped

6 bay leaves

Light spray of olive oil

Sea salt and freshly ground black pepper (to taste)

*Use coconut aminos for a soy-free alternative.

1. In a medium saucepan, combine the water, chicken, soy sauce, vinegar, garlic, and bay leaves. Bring to a boil over medium-high heat. Reduce the heat to medium-low and simmer, uncovered to allow the broth to reduce, for 35 minutes, stirring occasionally.

2. Lightly spray a nonstick skillet with olive oil. Using tongs, transfer the chicken from the saucepan to the skillet. Place the skillet over high heat and sauté to brown the chicken. Add 4 to 5 tablespoons of the broth

from the pot to the skillet, cover, and cook for about 90 seconds. Flip the chicken pieces and cook for an additional 90 seconds, until meat is visibly browned. Remove from the heat.

3. Meanwhile, continue to reduce the liquid in the saucepan over high heat for 8 to 10 minutes, until the sauce is thickened slightly and reduced to about half the original amount. Pour the sauce into a small storage container for ease of pouring over cooked meat.

4. Pour about ¼ cup of the reduced sauce over the chicken in the skillet, then transfer contents to a serving platter or shallow, microwave-safe, resealable dish. Serve hot right away, or allow the contents to cool at room temperature for 20 minutes before refrigerating.

Meal Prep Tips
- Store as a bulk protein source for variety if you do not wish to preportion out every single meal. Keeps for 4 days refrigerated.
- You can turn the chicken into a fatty protein for the meal plans by keeping the chicken skin on the thighs or legs.

Macros per 4-ounce serving:
Calories (kCal) 180; Total Fat 9g (Saturated Fat 3g, Trans Fat 0g); Cholesterol 75mg; Sodium 760mg; Potassium 360mg; Total Carbohydrate 5g (Dietary Fiber 0g, Sugars 3g); Protein 19g

Blueberry-Almond French Toast Protein Bake

Serves 6
Prep Time: 10 minutes, plus at least 20 minutes (or overnight) refrigeration
Cook Time: 40 minutes
MEAL PLAN KEY: LEAN PROTEIN + HIGH-GI CARB

If you are looking for a convenient meal that you can prepare in advance, this protein-packed baked French toast is easier than it looks — and completely filling and satisfying. Most French toast recipes are loaded with carbs and fat and lacking in protein. This healthy version is great for preparing in bulk or for feeding a crowd for a healthy brunch or family breakfast!

Ingredients

6 slices gluten-free bread*

8 oz (1 cup) frozen blueberries**

4 oz (4 scoops) vanilla-flavored whey protein isolate

8 oz (1 cup) egg whites*** (from about 8 large eggs)

8 oz (1 cup) unsweetened almond milk

1 teaspoon vanilla extract

1 teaspoon baking powder

2 teaspoons ground cinnamon

2 teaspoons sliced almonds, for garnish (optional)

I use Trader Joe's gluten-free bread.

*** Instead of blueberries, you can substitute strawberries, raspberries, blackberries, or a mix of berries.*

**** For convenience, I use liquid egg whites in the carton (found in the refrigerated dairy section of grocery stores). You can also separate whole eggs.*

1. Cut the bread into quarters, and then quarter them again to create cubes. Place in a 9-inch nonstick pie dish and sprinkle the blueberries on top.

2. In a bowl, combine the whey protein, egg whites, almond milk, vanilla extract, and baking powder. Mix well with a hand mixer, immersion blender, or shaker cup. Pour the egg white mixture over the bread and blueberries, and sprinkle the cinnamon evenly across the top. Refrigerate for at least 30 minutes or up to overnight to allow the bread cubes to soak up the egg.

3. When you're ready to bake it, preheat the oven to 350°F. Bake the French toast for 40 minutes, until risen, firmed up, and lightly browned.

4. Garnish with the sliced almonds before serving, if desired.

Meal Prep Tips

- Great for meal planning breakfast in bulk.
- Baked leftovers keep for 4 days, refrigerated.
- Leftovers can be enjoyed cold or reheated in a toaster oven for 60 seconds, a microwave for 30 seconds, or an air fryer for 2 to 3 minutes.

Macros per serving:

Calories (kCal) 281; Total Fat 3g (Saturated Fat 0g, Trans Fat 0g); Cholesterol 0mg; Sodium 441mg; Potassium 451mg; Total Carbohydrate 29g (Dietary Fiber 3g, Sugars 8g); Protein 34g

Simple Protein Waffles

Makes 1 serving

Prep Time: 10 minutes

Cook Time: 10 minutes

MEAL PLAN KEY: LEAN PROTEIN + HIGH-GI CARB

Mastering the formula for high-protein living includes learning how to enjoy old favorites like waffles and pancakes without blowing your carb budget for the day. This simple batter works well as waffles or pancakes. Add the toppings of your choice to take it to the next level.

Ingredients

1 oz (1 scoop) vanilla-flavored whey protein isolate

4 oz (½ cup) egg whites (from about 4 eggs)

2 oz (¼ cup) water

1.5 oz (½ cup) instant dry oats

¼ teaspoon baking powder

Oil spray of your choice

1. Combine the whey protein, egg whites, water, oats, and baking powder in a blender and blend until smooth.

2. To make waffles, lightly spray a waffle iron with oil spray and heat until griddle is ready. Spoon 2 to 3 tablespoons of the batter onto the waffle iron to make mini waffles, and cook according to manufacturer's directions. You can also make one big waffle.

3. To make pancakes, lightly coat a nonstick skillet or griddle with oil spray and heat over medium heat. Spoon the batter onto the skillet or griddle to desired pancake size and cook for 1 to 2 minutes, until pancakes bubble

and edges appear to have firmed up. Flip the pancakes and cook for another minute or so, until batter is cooked.

4. If making mini waffles or pancakes, work in batches and lightly coat the waffle iron, skillet, or griddle as needed with oil spray.

Macros per serving:
Calories (kCal) 320; Total Fat 3g (Saturated Fat 1g, Trans Fat 0g); Cholesterol 0mg; Sodium 340mg; Potassium 420mg; Total Carbohydrate 32g (Dietary Fiber 4g, Sugars 1g); Protein 43g

Thai-Style Basil Chicken

Makes 8 servings
Prep Time: 10 minutes, plus 30 minutes (or up to overnight) for marinating
Cook Time: 15 minutes
MEAL PLAN KEY: LEAN PROTEIN

This spicy chicken is the perfect solution when you want a healthier version of takeout. Don't skimp on the dried chile peppers — the seeds take the chicken to another level of heat if you enjoy authentic spice.

Ingredients
1 oz (2 tablespoons) olive oil
2 oz (¼ cup) distilled white vinegar
2 oz (¼ cup) soy sauce*
4 dried bird's beak chile peppers, sliced
5 cloves garlic, chopped
3 tablespoons chopped basil
32 oz (2 lb) boneless skinless chicken breast
Additional basil, for garnish (optional)
Use coconut aminos for a soy-free alternative

1. In a gallon freezer bag, combine 1 tablespoon of the olive oil and all the remaining ingredients except the chicken. Mix the marinade thoroughly, then add the chicken to the bag and shake well. Marinate at room temperature for 30 minutes or refrigerate overnight.

2. Heat the remaining 1 tablespoon olive oil in a large skillet over medium-high heat. Add the chicken breasts and the marinade and cook, turning the chicken once, for 4 minutes. Remove the chicken from the skillet and set on a cutting board. Slice chicken into strips where the inside is still pink.

3. Return the still-pink chicken slices to the skillet and cook on the flat sides until the juices brown the meat, about 1 minute per side. Continue this process until all of the chicken is thoroughly cooked but still juicy.

4. Allow 5 minutes for chicken to cool and then garnish with additional basil.

Macros per 4-ounce serving:
Calories (kCal) 137; Total Fat 4g (Saturated Fat 1g, Trans Fat 0g); Cholesterol 65mg; Sodium 841mg; Potassium 14mg; Total Carbohydrate 2g (Dietary Fiber 0g, Sugars 1g); Protein 24g

Cantaloupe-Kale-Chia Protein Shake

Makes 1 serving
Prep Time: 10 minutes
Cook Time: none
MEAL PLAN KEY: LEAN PROTEIN + LOW-GI CARB

When you need to replenish your body with dense nutrients, this protein shake is the answer. Loaded with superfoods that will leave you energized, detoxified, and rehydrated, it's a terrific post-workout drink or meal replacer. It deserves bonus points because it also supports healthy skin and boosts digestion.

Ingredients
1 oz (1 scoop) vanilla-flavored whey protein isolate
3 oz (½ cup) cubed cantaloupe
1 oz (1 cup) kale, stemmed
1 tablespoon chia seeds
8 oz (1 cup) water
Ice (optional)

1. Combine all ingredients in a blender and blend on high for 15 to 30 seconds until well mixed.

2. Pour into a large glass or mason jar with ice, and enjoy!

Macros per serving:

Calories (kCal) 206; Total Fat 3g (Saturated Fat 1g, Trans Fat 0g); Cholesterol 0mg; Sodium 118mg; Potassium 694mg; Total Carbohydrate 15g (Dietary Fiber 6g, Sugars 7g); Protein 30g

Mixed Berry–Almond Protein Shake

Makes 1 serving
Prep Time: 3 minutes
Cook Time: none
MEAL PLAN KEY: LEAN PROTEIN + LOW-GI CARB

I am a creature of habit, and once I came across this ingredient combination, I had the shake as my post-workout meal for almost two years straight. I'm a huge fan of frozen mixed berries. You never need to worry about them going bad, and they are a wonderful low-sugar post-workout carb source to replenish your tired muscles!

Ingredients

1 oz (1 scoop) vanilla-flavored whey protein isolate
2 oz (¼ cup) frozen mixed berries
8 oz (1 cup) unsweetened almond milk
1 teaspoon almond extract
Ice (optional)

1. Combine all ingredients in a blender and blend on high for 15 to 30 seconds until well mixed.

2. Pour into a large glass or mason jar with ice, and enjoy!

Macros per serving:

Calories (kCal) 173; Total Fat 4g (Saturated Fat 0g, Trans Fat 0g); Cholesterol 0mg; Sodium 178mg; Potassium 275mg; Total Carbohydrate 7g (Dietary Fiber 2g, Sugars 3g); Protein 26g

Chocolate-Coconut Cake Batter Protein Shake

Makes 1 serving

Prep Time: 3 minutes

Cook Time: none

MEAL PLAN KEY: LEAN PROTEIN + LOW-GI CARB

Every time a client asks me what to do to curb sugar cravings during that time of the month, I always point them in the direction of chocolate protein shakes. The natural sweetness of quality protein powder paired with unsweetened cocoa creates a rich, creamy, and satisfying flavor without throwing you off track. Experience a new way to satisfy cravings that doesn't involve sabotaging your progress!

Ingredients

1 oz (1 scoop) chocolate-flavored whey protein isolate

0.8 oz (3 tablespoons) unsweetened cocoa powder

8 oz (1 cup) unsweetened coconut milk

1 teaspoon maple extract

Ice (optional)

1. Combine all ingredients in a blender and blend on high for 15 to 30 seconds until well mixed.
2. Pour into a large glass or mason jar with ice, and enjoy!

Macros per serving:

Calories (kCal) 191; Total Fat 7g (Saturated Fat 5g, Trans Fat 0g); Cholesterol 0mg; Sodium 123mg; Potassium 486mg; Total Carbohydrate 13g (Dietary Fiber 7g, Sugars 0g); Protein 28g

Antioxidant Detox Smoothie

Makes 1 serving

Prep Time: 3 minutes

Cook Time: none

MEAL PLAN KEY: LEAN PROTEIN + HIGH-GI CARB

This shake is wonderful if you are just getting back on track from a hiatus from your nutrition plan or if you recently drank excess alcohol. Naturally detoxifying kale and flaxseeds support healthy digestion and restore vitamins and minerals.

Ingredients

1 oz (1 scoop) vanilla-flavored whey protein isolate

2 oz (¼ cup) blueberries

2 oz (¼ cup) sliced apples

1 oz (1 cup) kale, de-stemmed

1 tablespoon flaxseeds

8 oz (1 cup) unsweetened coconut milk

Ice (optional)

1. Combine all ingredients in a blender and blend on high for 15 to 30 seconds until well mixed.
2. Pour into a large glass or mason jar with ice, and enjoy!

Macros per serving:

Calories (kCal) 239; Total Fat 8g (Saturated Fat 4g, Trans Fat 0g); Cholesterol 0mg; Sodium 132mg; Potassium 408mg; Total Carbohydrate 17g (Dietary Fiber 5g, Sugars 7g); Protein 28g

Blueberry-Watermelon Post-Workout Shake

Makes 1 serving

Prep Time: 3 minutes

Cook Time: none

MEAL PLAN KEY: LEAN PROTEIN + HIGH-GI CARB

This shake is a must when you need to replace electrolytes from a hard workout. Watermelon is naturally high in electrolytes as well as citrulline malate, an ingredient known for its recovery-boosting properties.

Ingredients

　　1 oz (1 scoop) vanilla-flavored whey protein isolate

　　5.4 oz (1 cup) cubed watermelon

　　2 oz (¼ cup) blueberries

　　8 oz (1 cup) water

　　Ice (optional)

1. Combine all ingredients in a blender and blend on high for 15 to 30 seconds until well mixed.
2. Pour into a large glass or mason jar with ice, and enjoy!

Macros per serving:

　　Calories (kCal) 177; Total Fat 0g (Saturated Fat 0g, Trans Fat 0g); Cholesterol 0mg; Sodium 82mg; Potassium 439mg; Total Carbohydrate 19g (Dietary Fiber 2g, Sugars 13g); Protein 26g

Chocolate Pretzel Protein Shake

Makes 1 serving

Prep Time: 3 minutes

Cook Time: none

MEAL PLAN KEY: LEAN PROTEIN + LOW-GI CARB

If you find yourself getting bored with your post-workout routine, mix it up with this delicious sweet-and-salty combination of chocolate and pretzels. Excellent for when you are craving chocolate and sweets.

Ingredients

　　1 oz (1 scoop) chocolate-flavored whey protein isolate

　　0.6 oz (2 tablespoons) unsweetened cocoa powder

　　0.3 oz (1 tablespoon) chocolate chips

　　4 mini pretzels

　　¼ teaspoon sea salt

　　8 oz (1 cup) water

　　½ cup ice

1. Combine all ingredients in a blender and blend on high for 15 to 30 seconds until well mixed.
2. Pour into a large glass or mason jar with ice, and enjoy!

Macros per serving:
Calories (kCal) 215; Total Fat 5g (Saturated Fat 3g, Trans Fat 0g); Cholesterol 0mg; Sodium 672mg; Potassium 404mg; Total Carbohydrate 19g (Dietary Fiber 5g, Sugars 8g); Protein 28g

Strawberry-Pineapple Protein Shake

Makes 1 serving
Prep Time: 3 minutes
Cook Time: none
MEAL PLAN KEY: LEAN PROTEIN + LOW-GI CARB

Replenish tired muscles with this simple, yet fresh tropical smoothie that is packed with flavor and loaded with nutrients. Pineapples contain the enzyme bromelain, which is not only great for reducing inflammation and promoting recovery, but it also boosts the uptake of protein. When combined with strawberries, which are high in electrolytes, this makes for a nutrient-dense, functional shake that you will absolutely love!

Ingredients
1 oz (1 scoop) vanilla-flavored whey protein isolate
2 oz (¼ cup) sliced strawberries
2 oz (¼ cup) diced pineapple
8 oz (1 cup) unsweetened almond milk
1 teaspoon almond extract
Ice (optional)

1. Combine all ingredients in a blender and blend on high for 15 to 30 seconds until well mixed.
2. Pour into a large glass or mason jar with ice, and enjoy!

Macros per serving:

Calories (kCal) 177; Total Fat 3g (Saturated Fat 0g, Trans Fat 0g); Cholesterol 0mg; Sodium 240mg; Potassium 372mg; Total Carbohydrate 12g (Dietary Fiber 1g, Sugars 4g); Protein 25g

Fatty Protein Recipes

Chimichurri Chicken Thighs

Makes 10 thighs
Prep Time: 15 minutes
Cook Time: 50 minutes
MEAL PLAN KEY: FATTY PROTEIN

Enjoy this budget-friendly chicken that is crispy, flavorful, and healthy! I'm obsessed with chicken thighs because they just taste so good and are way more affordable than other protein sources. If you are trying to lose weight, the key to making this recipe work in a lower-fat meal plan is to balance out your macros for your goals. For example, if your total daily fat intake goal is only 50 grams per day, one serving would take almost half of your total daily fat intake, so be aware of how that impacts your choices outside of a meal including this recipe. These thighs are a family favorite and are great for serving a crowd without breaking the bank.

Ingredients

Coconut oil or olive oil spray
10 bone-in chicken thighs with skin

CHIMICHURRI
0.8 oz (1½ cups) chopped cilantro
1.8 oz (½ cup) chopped Italian parsley
2 oz (¼ cup) extra-virgin olive oil
2 oz (¼ cup) distilled white vinegar

2.1 oz (¼ cup) minced garlic

2 oz lime juice (juice of 2 large limes)

1 oz jalapeño, sliced (~1 small pepper)

5 teaspoons ground cumin, plus more to taste

3 teaspoons oregano

Sea salt and black pepper (to taste)

1. Preheat the oven to 425°F. Line a baking sheet with foil and lightly spray with coconut oil or olive oil spray.
2. Make the chimichurri: Combine all the chimichurri ingredients in a food processor and blend on low for 10 to 15 seconds.
3. For each chicken thigh, peel back the skin and place 1 tablespoon of the chimichurri under the skin. Place skin-side down on the prepared baking sheet. Spoon half of the remaining chimichurri over the thighs and then top with more cumin and sea salt.
4. Bake the chicken for 20 minutes. Remove the pan from the oven and pour off the excess liquid. Gently flip each piece of chicken over, season with more cumin and sea salt, and top with the rest of the chimichurri. Bake for 25 minutes, until skin is visibly browned.
5. Lightly spray the chicken with coconut or olive oil and broil for about 5 minutes (watching carefully), until the skin is browned and crispy. Let rest for 5 to 10 minutes before serving.

Meal Prep Tips
- Excellent family-friendly recipe to batch cook for a few days' worth of meals.
- Recommend using an air fryer to reheat cooked thighs for 2 to 3 minutes at 370°F, a microwave for 1 minute 30 seconds on high, or broil in an oven for 2 minutes.
- Cooked chicken thighs keep in the fridge for 3 to 4 days or in the freezer for up to 2 months.

Macros per 4-ounce thigh with skin and bone:
  Calories (kCal) 308; Total Fat 23g (Saturated Fat 6g, Trans Fat 0g); Cholesterol 95mg;
  Sodium 331mg; Potassium 125mg; Total Carbohydrate 4g (Dietary Fiber 1g, Sugars 0g);
  Protein 20g

Slow-Cooker Pork Carnitas

Makes 16 servings

Prep Time: 15 minutes

Cook Time: 6 hours

MEAL PLAN KEY: FATTY PROTEIN

This recipe is the best thing that has ever been made in my slow cooker, like ever. The amazing combination of subtle spices provides a rich flavor that penetrates the pork, which then shreds effortlessly with a fork after slow cooking. Carnitas are the perfect meal that can be served as a taco, salad, with veggies or the carb of your choice and are great when cooking for a budget-conscious household.

Ingredients
  64 oz (4 lb) pork butt
  3 oz lime juice (juice of 3 large limes)
  2.35 oz (½ cup) cumin
  2 oz jalapeños, seeded and chopped
  5 oz (~1 medium) red onion, chopped
  2 tablespoons dried oregano
  1 tablespoon dried thyme
  2 tablespoons cayenne pepper
  2 tablespoons sea salt
  Chopped fresh cilantro for garnish (optional)

1. Place the pork in the slow cooker and top with two-thirds of the lime juice (from 2 limes), ¼ cup of the cumin, the jalapeños, onion, oregano, and thyme. Cover, set to low, and cook for 6 hours.

2. After 6 hours, turn the slow cooker off, and use tongs to carefully transfer the pork to a large mixing bowl, reserving the juices in the cooker. Carefully shred the pork using two forks. Pour all of the juice from the slow cooker over the meat.

3. Add the remaining lime juice, remaining ¼ cup cumin, the cayenne, and salt to the shredded meat and mix thoroughly until fully incorporated.

4. Allow to cool before serving. Top with cilantro as an optional garnish.

Macros per 4-ounce serving:
Calories (kCal) 319; Total Fat 22g (Saturated Fat 6g, Trans Fat 0g); Cholesterol 97mg; Sodium 966mg; Potassium 447mg; Total Carbohydrate 2g (Dietary Fiber 1g, Sugars 1g); Protein 27g

Italian Meatballs

Makes 20 meatballs
Prep Time: 20 minutes
Cook Time: 25 minutes
MEAL PLAN KEY: FATTY PROTEIN

Meatballs are the ultimate comfort food for many families. This is a healthy makeover of a classic, with a flavorful blend of herbal spices and a cooking method that yields the most tender meatballs you have ever had in your life. Eating healthy doesn't mean eating dry, lifeless foods any longer! You can substitute ground turkey or chicken for the ground beef for a lower-fat recipe that is equally delicious. Serve over cooked spaghetti squash, zucchini, or the starches of your choice for an alternative to pasta.

Ingredients
Olive oil spray

MEATBALLS
16 oz (1 lb) 80 percent ground beef
3.5 oz (½ cup) Italian parsley

2 tablespoons grated Parmesan cheese

4 cloves garlic, minced

4 teaspoons dried oregano

4 teaspoons dried thyme

1 teaspoon black pepper

1 teaspoon red pepper flakes

Sea salt (to taste)

MARINARA SAUCE

1 (15-oz) can salt-free diced tomatoes, drained

2 oz (¼ cup) extra-virgin olive oil

2 cloves garlic

1 tablespoon oregano

1 teaspoon black pepper

¼ teaspoon sea salt

1. Preheat the oven to 375°F. Line a baking sheet with foil and lightly spray with olive oil spray, or line with parchment paper, and set aside.
2. Make the meatballs: In a large mixing bowl, thoroughly combine the meatball ingredients until well mixed. Form meatballs by rolling in the palms of your hands, using about 1 tablespoon of meat per meatball.
3. Place on prepared baking sheet and bake for 25 minutes, until texture is firm and outer surface is browned.
4. Meanwhile, make the marinara: Combine all the marinara ingredients in a food processor and process until garlic and herbs are fully distributed. Heat the marinara in a large skillet over medium heat.
5. Add the meatballs and thoroughly cover with sauce. Cover and simmer for 1 to 2 minutes, until sauce is absorbed into the meatballs.

Macros per 2 meatballs with sauce:
Calories (kCal) 160; Total Fat 12g (Saturated Fat 4g, Trans Fat 0g); Cholesterol 44mg; Sodium 540mg; Potassium 266mg; Total Carbohydrate 4g (Dietary Fiber 0g, Sugars 2g); Protein 22g

Salmon with Parmesan and Garlic-Rosemary Butter

Makes 2 servings
Prep Time: 20 minutes
Cook Time: 25 to 30 minutes
MEAL PLAN KEY: FATTY PROTEIN

If I could eat one protein source every day for the rest of my life, it would be salmon. This recipe is hands-down one of my all-time favorites — I never get tired of these rich, healthy, and delicious flavors. If you want to take your cooking to the next level, make this for yourself and enjoy the crispy finish on top of the delicate and juicy tenderness of the salmon.

Ingredients

Butter spray or olive oil spray
2 (4-oz) wild salmon fillets
Sea salt and black pepper (to taste)
2 tablespoons Garlic-Rosemary Butter (see page 263)
1.59 oz (½ cup) grated Parmesan cheese

1. Preheat the oven to 350°F. Line a baking sheet with foil and spray with butter or olive oil spray.
2. Place the salmon on the lined baking sheet and season with salt and pepper. Drop 1 tablespoon Garlic-Rosemary Butter on each piece of salmon and wrap together in the foil. Bake for 15 minutes. Open foil to expose the salmon. Sprinkle each piece of salmon with ¼ cup Parmesan. Return to the oven and bake, uncovered, for 3 to 5 more minutes, until cheese is melted and turned to a light golden brown color.
3. Set the oven to broil for 4 to 5 minutes and cook until cheese is lightly browned and crispy on the edges. Remove from oven and cool for 5 to 10 minutes before serving.

Macros per 1 salmon fillet w/topping:
Calories (kCal) 352; Total Fat 23g (Saturated Fat 12g, Trans Fat 0g); Cholesterol 105mg; Sodium 693mg; Potassium 7mg; Total Carbohydrate 0.4g (Dietary Fiber 0g, Sugars 0g); Protein 33g

Hummus Deviled Eggs

Makes 12 servings
Prep Time: 10 minutes
Cook Time: 15 minutes
MEAL PLAN KEY: FATTY PROTEIN

Enjoy this incredibly delicious recipe that only requires three ingredients: eggs, hummus, and bacon! This is a favorite appetizer at parties and an incredibly rich and flavorful lower-fat alternative to traditional deviled eggs. You can experiment with different hummus flavors for added variety to this simple recipe!

Ingredients
4 slices bacon
6 hard-boiled eggs, peeled
4.5 oz (½ cup) hummus (flavor and brand of your choice)
Sea salt and black pepper (to taste)

1. Panfry the bacon in a skillet until crisp, and let cool. Crumble by chopping with a knife or by breaking up by hand.
2. Cut the peeled eggs lengthwise in half and scoop out the yolks and discard.
3. Add 2 teaspoons hummus to each halved egg. Season with sea salt and black pepper to taste. Top with crumbled bacon and enjoy!

Macros per ½ egg:
Calories (kCal) 76g; Total Fat 6g (Saturated Fat 0g, Trans Fat 0g); Cholesterol 96g; Sodium 128g; Potassium 45g; Total Carbohydrate 2g (Dietary Fiber 1g, Sugar 1g); Protein 5g

Garlic and Mushroom White Pizza

Makes 8 slices
Prep Time: 20 minutes
Cook Time: 25 minutes
MEAL PLAN KEY: FATTY PROTEIN

The words *pizza* and *carbs* are almost synonymous. So you can imagine my boyfriend's surprise when I first created this recipe for him a few years ago. He's a picky eater, so I made the pizza and said nothing. He loved it and ate the entire thing in a single sitting. He was shocked when I told him there are more carbs in a small apple than in the entire pizza! That's when I knew this recipe was a hit. Bake one up when you need a delicious low-carb meal or when you need to serve a healthy meal to someone who refuses "diet food."

Ingredients

PIZZA CRUST

4.4 oz (1 cup) frozen cauliflower rice

2.0 oz (½ cup) shredded full-fat mozzarella cheese

1.5 oz (½ cup) grated Parmesan cheese

1 large egg

PIZZA TOPPINGS

4 cloves garlic, peeled

1 oz (3 tablespoons) extra-virgin olive oil

4 oz (1 cup) shredded full-fat mozzarella cheese

1 oz (¼ cup) sliced portabella mushrooms

Sea salt (to taste)

Black pepper (to taste)

Fresh basil (optional)

Cauliflower Pizza Crust Recipe

1. Make the crust: Preheat the oven to 400°F. Line a baking sheet with parchment paper.

2. Evenly spread the frozen riced cauliflower in a large bowl up and along the sides of the bowl (to allow maximum water to escape). Microwave on high for 5 minutes, until cauliflower appears to be visibly dried out. Add the mozzarella, Parmesan, and egg and mix by hand.

3. Flatten the "dough" on the lined baking sheet. Be careful to not spread so thin that holes form. Note that it will not feel the same as a traditional

flour-based dough. Rather, it will feel like a hash brown but will become solid as it bakes. Bake for 10 to 15 minutes, and remove from oven. Set aside until you are ready to make pizza.

4. Make the pizza: Preheat the oven to 400°F.

5. Slice the garlic lengthwise and lay flat on the pizza crust. Paint the garlic with 1 tablespoon of the olive oil. Top with the mozzarella cheese.

6. Heat the remaining 2 tablespoons oil in a skillet over medium-high heat. Add the mushrooms and sauté for 1 minute. Place on top of pizza.

7. Bake the pizza for 10 to 12 minutes, until the cheese is melted and the crust is lightly toasted. Season with salt and pepper, and top with fresh basil if you like.

Macros per slice:
Calories (kCal) 136; Total Fat 10g (Saturated Fat 4g, Trans Fat 0g); Cholesterol 43mg; Sodium 266mg; Potassium 57mg; Total Carbohydrate 2g (Dietary Fiber 0.4g, Sugars 0g); Protein 9 g

Macros per 1 pizza crust:
Calories (kCal) 496; Total Fat 31g (Saturated Fat 17g, Trans Fat 0g); Cholesterol 275mg; Sodium 1,037mg; Potassium 305mg; Total Carbohydrate 10g (Dietary Fiber 3g, Sugars 3g); Protein 43g

Chicken Sausage and Cauliflower Stuffing

Makes 8 servings
Prep Time: 10 minutes
Cook Time: 15 minutes
MEAL PLAN KEY: FATTY PROTEIN

If you miss traditional bread-based side dishes like stuffing on your holiday table, your longing ends today. This stuffing recipe is light, delicious, and packed with flavor — without loading you down with carbs. Enjoy this lightened-up stuffing that makes an excellent side — or main dish — any time of year!

Ingredients

SEASONED SAUSAGE

Olive oil spray

16 oz (1 lb) chicken sausage links

1 tablespoon extra-virgin olive oil

3 cloves garlic, minced

1 tablespoon dried thyme

1 tablespoon paprika

1 teaspoon black pepper

¼ teaspoon sea salt

"STUFFING"

4 tablespoons extra-virgin olive oil

16 oz (4 cups) riced cauliflower*

4 oz (3 stalks) celery

5 oz (~2 whole sticks) carrots

4 oz (½ cup) chicken stock

You can find frozen, pre-riced cauliflower in the frozen foods aisle, or get a large head of cauliflower and rice it in a food processor.

1. Cook the sausage: Spray a nonstick skillet lightly with olive oil. Add the sausage and cook over medium-high heat for 2 minutes per side; set aside. Slice the sausages into ½-inch pieces.

2. Add the olive oil to the skillet and sauté the garlic over medium-high heat for 30 to 45 seconds, until softened. Add the sliced sausage, thyme, paprika, pepper, and salt and sauté for 3 to 5 minutes, until the sausage pieces are lightly browned and cooked through.

3. Make the stuffing: In a separate large skillet, heat the olive oil over medium-high heat. Add the riced cauliflower, celery, and carrots and cook for 2 to 3 minutes. Add the seasoned sausage and stock and stir for 30 to 60 more seconds, until the stock has cooked down and evaporated. Remove from heat and cool for 3 minutes, then fluff and serve.

Macros per ¾-cup serving:
   Calories (kCal) 230; Total Fat 12g (Saturated Fat 3g, Trans Fat 0g); Cholesterol 71mg;
   Sodium 307mg; Potassium 312mg; Total Carbohydrate 7g (Dietary Fiber 2g, Sugars 3g);
   Protein 23g

Spaghetti Squash Pizza Casserole

Makes 4 servings

Prep Time: 40 minutes (including roasting squash)

Cook Time: 20 minutes

MEAL PLAN KEY: FATTY PROTEIN + LOW-GI CARB

When you are committed to healthy living but still need delicious food that will satisfy the whole family, this dish is a go-to! Experience all the tasty flavors of pizza with only one-third of the carb content. The recipe is not only easy and satisfying, but it can also be customized to include your favorite low-calorie, high-flavor toppings like hot peppers, veggies, and greens.

Ingredients
   Olive oil spray
   17.6 oz (4 cups) spaghetti squash* (~½ medium)
   3.5 oz (½ cup) canned diced tomatoes
   2 whole large eggs
   1 tablespoon dried oregano
   1 tablespoon garlic powder
   ¼ teaspoon sea salt
   6 oz (about 1½ cups) shredded mozzarella cheese
   1.3 oz (about ½ cup) sliced portabella mushrooms
   12 slices pepperoni**
   2 tablespoons black olives

* *To halve spaghetti squash, carefully score the squash around the perimeter and slice in half lengthwise with a large knife. You can also microwave the squash for about 2 to 3 minutes to make it easier to cut in half.*

** *You can use organic turkey pepperoni for a pork-free alternative.*

1. Preheat the oven to 350°F. Line a baking sheet with parchment paper. Lightly spray an 8 × 8-inch nonstick baking dish with olive oil.

2. Scoop out the seeds from the squash half with a spoon. Lightly spray the squash half with olive oil and place cut-side down on the lined baking sheet. Roast for 35 to 40 minutes, until softened. Allow the squash to cool for 2 to 3 minutes. Using a fork, scrape out the insides and reserve the long spaghetti-like strands of squash. You should have about 3 cups. Discard the empty rind.

3. Spread the squash strands evenly on the bottom of the prepared baking dish.

4. In a separate small mixing bowl, whisk together the tomatoes, eggs, oregano, garlic powder, and salt. Pour over the spaghetti squash. Top with mozzarella, mushrooms, pepperoni, and olives.

5. Bake for 20 minutes. Set to broil and broil for 1 to 2 minutes. Let cool for 5 minutes before serving.

Macros per serving:
Calories (kCal) 249; Total Fat 15g (Saturated Fat 7g, Trans Fat 0g); Cholesterol 130mg; Sodium 1,063mg; Potassium 185mg; Total Carbohydrate 13g (Dietary Fiber 2g, Sugars 8g); Protein 15g

Cheddar-Jalapeño Cauliflower Biscuits

Makes 10 servings
Prep Time: 15 minutes
Cook Time: 20 minutes
MEAL PLAN KEY: FATTY PROTEIN (4 BISCUITS)

I've shared this recipe with my clients, and they never fail to tell me that these low-carb delights actually taste like real biscuits. With only 1 gram of net carbs per serving, the biscuits are an amazing addition to your low-carb lifestyle. The easy recipe allows you to stay on track with your goals with just the right amount of kick from jalapeño and rich savory flavor from cheddar.

Ingredients

    16 oz (4¼ cups) cauliflower florets

    4 oz (1 cup) shredded sharp cheddar cheese, plus 1.73 oz (10 tea-
        spoons) for topping

    3 large eggs

    1 oz jalapeño, sliced

    ½ teaspoon sea salt

    ¼ teaspoon black pepper

    ¼ teaspoon baking powder

1. Preheat the oven to 400°F. Line a baking sheet with parchment paper and set aside.

2. Combine all the ingredients in a food processor and process on high for 1 minute, or until thoroughly mixed to a consistency resembling thick oatmeal or mashed potatoes.

3. Using a ¼-cup measuring cup, scoop the batter onto the baking sheet to make about 10 biscuits. Top each with about 1 teaspoon shredded cheddar cheese. Bake for about 20 minutes, until firm with a light golden-brown color. Broil for 30 seconds until golden brown. Let cool for 10 minutes before serving.

Macros per serving:

    Calories (kCal) 67; Total Fat 5g (Saturated Fat 2g, Trans Fat 0g); Cholesterol 67mg; Sodium 335mg; Potassium 88mg; Total Carbohydrate 2g (Dietary Fiber 1g, Sugars 1g); Protein 5g

Grilled Sausage-Stuffed Delicata Squash Boats

Makes 8 servings
Prep Time: 25 minutes
Cook Time: 30 minutes
MEAL PLAN KEY: FATTY PROTEIN

It's easy to fall into a rut on a lower-carb meal plan, eating the same vegetables over and over. If this is you, try mixing it up with sausage-stuffed squash boats. Experience filling flavor, variety, and a wonderful low-carb meal that will keep you on track without a ton of fuss!

Ingredients

16 oz hot Italian sausages, casings removed

2 oz (2 cups) spinach

48 oz (~4 medium) delicata squash

4 oz (1 cup) gorgonzola cheese crumbles

Sea salt and black pepper (to taste)

1. Preheat a grill to medium (or the oven to 350°F).
2. Heat a nonstick skillet over medium-high heat. Add the sausage and cook for 5 minutes, using a spatula to break it into crumbled ground meat. Press the spatula over the sausage crumbles and tilt the pan to drain the excess fat from the pan. Continue to cook the sausage for 2 to 3 minutes, until browned. Add the spinach and stir-fry for 30 to 60 seconds, until wilted.
3. Slice each squash in half lengthwise and scrape out the seeds. Spoon the crumbled sausage and spinach evenly into the squash boats and top with the gorgonzola cheese.
4. Grill over medium heat (or bake on a parchment-lined baking sheet) for 15 to 20 minutes, until the squash is softened and the cheese is melted. Season with sea salt and pepper to taste.

Macros per squash boat:

Calories (kCal) 321; Total Fat 21g (Saturated Fat 8g, Trans Fat 0g); Cholesterol 58mg; Sodium 766mg; Potassium 779mg; Total Carbohydrate 20g (Dietary Fiber 3g, Sugars 4g); Protein 16g

Feta and Red Pepper Vegetarian Quiche

Makes 6 servings

Prep Time: 5 minutes

Cook Time: 30 minutes

MEAL PLAN KEY: FATTY PROTEIN

If you are a fan of savory breakfasts, this feta-based quiche will quickly become a new favorite. Not only is it easy to make, but the quiche also reheats well for an easy lunch or simple dinner. It's an ideal recipe for batch cooking and a creative way to enjoy eggs on a lower-carb, higher-fat diet.

Ingredients
- Olive oil spray
- 6 large eggs
- 8.5 oz (1 cup) heavy whipping cream
- 2 teaspoons dried rosemary
- 2 teaspoons dried thyme
- 1 teaspoon black pepper
- Sea salt (to taste)
- 1 medium red bell pepper, cored, seeded, and chopped
- 2 oz (2 cups) spinach, chopped
- 4 oz (¾ cup) crumbled feta cheese

1. Preheat oven to 375°F. Lightly spray a 9-inch pie pan with olive oil spray and set aside.
2. In a large bowl, whisk together the eggs, cream, rosemary, thyme, pepper, and salt. Add the red pepper, spinach, and feta and stir to blend. Pour into the prepared pie pan.
3. Bake for about 30 minutes, until the quiche is set. Let cool for 10 minutes before serving.

Macros per serving:
Calories (kCal) 255; Total Fat 20g (Saturated Fat 11g, Trans Fat 0g); Cholesterol 245mg; Sodium 749mg; Potassium 210mg; Total Carbohydrate 4g (Dietary Fiber 1g, Sugars 2g); Protein 15g

Fatty Low-GI Carbs

Low-Carb Bread

Makes 10 servings

Prep Time: 15 minutes

Cook Time: 50 minutes

MEAL PLAN KEY: FATTY LOW-GI CARB

A higher-fat, lower-carb lifestyle enables stable energy without cravings for sugar. However, there are times when one simply misses the idea of carbs on an emotional level. With only 3 grams of net carbs, this "bread" is an incredibly moist, rich, flavorful, keto-friendly, low-carb treat without gluten or grains!

Ingredients

3 large eggs, separated

2 oz (¼ cup; 4 tablespoons) butter, melted (30 seconds in the microwave)

4 oz cream cheese, softened

5.1 oz (1½ cups) almond flour

1 tablespoon monk fruit (aka luo han guo) sweetener

2½ teaspoons baking soda

¼ teaspoon sea salt

1. Preheat the oven to 325°F. Line an 8½ × 4½-inch bread pan with parchment paper.
2. Whip the egg whites in a medium bowl with an immersion blender until a foamy consistency with a larger volume is achieved.
3. In a food processor, combine the egg yolks, melted butter, cream cheese, almond flour, sweetener, baking soda, and salt. Mix on low for 10 to 15 seconds, just until it becomes a smooth, creamy consistency. Be careful not to overmix. Add the whipped egg whites and mix for 5 to 10 seconds. Scrape the batter into the bread pan.

4. Bake for 50 minutes, until golden brown. Let cool for 20 minutes before removing from the pan. Enjoy!

Macros per serving:
   Calories (kCal) 166; Total Fat 16g (Saturated Fat 6g, Trans Fat 0g); Cholesterol 81mg; Sodium 344mg; Potassium 38mg; Total Carbohydrate 4g (Dietary Fiber 1g, Sugars 1g); Protein 5g

Creamy Brussels Sprouts Casserole

Makes 10 servings
Prep Time: 15 minutes
Cook Time: 30 minutes

MEAL PLAN KEY: FATTY LOW-GI CARB

If you have never been a fan of Brussels sprouts, all of that is about to change with one single bite of this *incredible* casserole. A unique blend of ingredients brings out a rich yet subtle sweetness in Brussels sprouts that you never knew existed. Say goodbye to bitter vegetables, and enjoy this remarkable side that your taste buds will never forget.

Ingredients
   Olive oil spray
   10 oz (2½ cups) shredded Brussels sprouts
   8 oz (2⅝ cups) sliced baby bella mushrooms
   1.4 oz (3 tablespoons) extra-virgin olive oil
   8 oz cream cheese, softened
   1 large egg
   1.59 oz (½ cup) grated Parmesan cheese
   Sea salt and black pepper (to taste)

1. Preheat the oven to 350°F. Lightly spray a 1.75-quart casserole dish with olive oil spray.
2. In a medium mixing bowl, combine the Brussels sprouts and mushrooms. Top with the olive oil and cream cheese and use a spoon to carefully blend the mixture. Add the egg and mix well.

3. Spoon the mixture into the casserole dish and top with the Parmesan cheese. Add salt and pepper to taste. Bake, uncovered, for 30 minutes at 350°F. Broil for 1 to 2 minutes to brown the top (optional). Cool for 3 to 5 minutes before serving.

Macros per ⅓-cup serving:
   Calories (kCal) 151; Total Fat 14g (Saturated Fat 6g, Trans Fat 0g); Cholesterol 47mg; Sodium 167mg; Potassium 180mg; Total Carbohydrate 3g (Dietary Fiber 1g, Sugars 1g); Protein 5g

Avocado Hummus

Makes about 10 servings
Prep Time: 10 minutes
Cook Time: none
MEAL PLAN KEY: FATTY LOW-GI CARB

You will never make or buy regular hummus again after you have tried this avocado-based recipe. The combination of avocado, chickpeas, and olive oil yields one of the creamiest, most delicious dips you will ever try. Pair with carrots, red peppers, celery, cucumbers, or other veggies of your choice!

Ingredients
   1 (15-oz) can chickpeas (garbanzo beans), drained and rinsed
   4 oz avocado
   Juice of 1 small lime
   0.57 oz (2 tablespoons) extra-virgin olive oil
   2 tablespoons ground cumin
   1 tablespoon garlic powder
   1 teaspoon paprika
   1 teaspoon sea salt
   ¼ teaspoon cayenne pepper

1. Blend all ingredients together in a food processor for 1 to 2 minutes, until it reaches a smooth yet creamy consistency.

2. Store in an airtight container until ready to use.

Macros per 2-tablespoon serving:
   Calories (kCal) 133; Total Fat 8g (Saturated Fat 1g, Trans Fat 0g); Cholesterol 0mg; Sodium 463mg; Potassium 114mg; Total Carbohydrate 6g (Dietary Fiber 1g, Sugars 0g); Protein 9g

Low-Carb Cauli Mac & Cheese

Makes 8 servings
Prep Time: 10 minutes
Cook Time: 10 minutes
MEAL PLAN KEY: FATTY LOW-GI CARB

Comfort food and carbs tend to go hand in hand. When you are on a lower-carb plan, the idea of saying goodbye to carbs forever is an awful thought. This recipe takes the goodness of mac and cheese and uses cauliflower as the base instead of macaroni for a wonderful, light, and extremely delicious treat with only 3 grams of net carbs per serving!

Ingredients
   5 slices bacon
   36 oz (2¼ lb) cauliflower florets
   4.2 oz (½ cup) heavy cream
   2 cloves garlic, minced
   4 oz (½ cup) shredded cheddar cheese
   4 oz (½ cup) shredded mozzarella cheese
   1 oz jalapeño, chopped
   1 teaspoon Dijon mustard powder (or other ground mustard powder)
   1 teaspoon paprika
   Sea salt and black pepper (to taste)

1. Preheat the oven to 450°F.
2. Panfry the bacon in a skillet and set aside. When cool, crumble by chopping with a knife or breaking up by hand.
3. Combine the cauliflower, cream, and garlic in a food processor and pulse for 10 to 15 seconds, until the cauliflower has a rice-like texture.
4. Transfer the riced cauliflower to a 13 × 9 × 2-inch baking pan. Sprinkle the bacon, cheddar, mozzarella, jalapeño, mustard powder, paprika, salt, and pepper over the cauliflower. Bake for 8 to 10 minutes, and then broil for 2 to 3 minutes to crisp up the top.

Macros per serving:
Calories (kCal) 150; Total Fat 12g (Saturated Fat 7g, Trans Fat 0g); Cholesterol 39mg; Sodium 227mg; Potassium 245mg; Total Carbs 5g (Dietary Fiber 2g, Sugars 2g); Protein 7g

Pumpkin Spice Keto Bread

Makes 10 servings
Prep Time: 15 minutes
Cook Time: 50 minutes
MEAL PLAN KEY: FATTY LOW-GI CARB

Pumpkin spice anything tends to be synonymous with a ton of added sugar. But you shouldn't have to skip seasonal favorites or feel deprived because of your health goals. The key is to rethink your foods and create new healthy favorites that are just as fun as the originals. This recipe is a wonderful staple for a low-carb lifestyle.

Ingredients
3 large eggs, separated
4 oz cream cheese, softened
2 oz (¼ cup, 4 tablespoons) butter, melted
1.64 oz (3 tablespoons) pumpkin puree
5.1 oz (1½ cups) almond flour

¼ cup monk fruit (aka luo han guo) sweetener

2 tablespoons pumpkin pie spice

1½ teaspoons baking soda

¼ teaspoon sea salt

1. Preheat the oven to 325°F. Line an 8½ × 4½-inch loaf pan with parchment paper.
2. Whip the egg whites in a medium bowl with an immersion blender into a foamy consistency with a larger volume.
3. In a food processor, combine the egg yolks, cream cheese, melted butter, pumpkin puree, almond flour, sweetener, pumpkin pie spice, baking soda, and salt. Mix on low for 10 to 15 seconds, just until batter turns into a smooth blended consistency. Be careful not to overmix.
4. Add the whipped egg whites and mix for 5 to 10 seconds.
5. Pour the batter into the loaf pan. Bake for 50 minutes, or until cooked through. Let cool for 20 minutes before removing from the pan. Enjoy!

Macros per serving:
Calories (kCal) 210; Total Fat 19g (Saturated Fat 6g, Trans Fat 0g); Cholesterol 81mg; Sodium 333mg; Potassium 60mg; Total Carbohydrate 10g (Dietary Fiber 1g, Sugars 1g); Protein 7g

Protein Snacks

Chocolate Chip Protein Blondies

Makes 16 servings
Prep Time: 10 minutes
Cook Time: 15 minutes
MEAL PLAN KEY: FATTY PROTEIN + LOW-GI CARB

The best part of these blondies is the fact that they don't just taste amazing, they are actually healthy for you. If you are a fan of chocolate chip cookies, you'll love this recipe because you won't feel deprived of your favorite baked goods. These decadent treats are a perfect snack or pre-workout pick-me-up when you are craving a healthy source of sweetness.

Ingredients

Coconut oil spray

12 oz mashed bananas (~3 large bananas)

8.5 oz (1 cup) almond butter (can use Toasted Coconut–Maple Almond Butter, page 267)

7 (1-gram) packets calorie-free sweetener of your choice*

2 teaspoons almond extract

Pinch of sea salt (optional)

4 oz (4 scoops) vanilla-flavored whey protein isolate

1.4 oz (¼ cup) chocolate chips

Examples include stevia and monk fruit (aka luo han guo) sweetener.

1. Preheat oven to 350°F. Spray a 9 × 9-inch nonstick baking pan with coconut oil.

2. Combine the mashed bananas, almond butter, sweetener, almond extract, and salt (optional) in a medium bowl. Mix well with a whisk or hand blender. Add the protein powder, one scoop at a time, mixing thoroughly between each scoop. Batter will have a smooth yet thick consistency.

3. Pour the batter into the prepared pan and sprinkle the chocolate chips over the top. Bake for about 15 minutes, until firm and golden brown.

4. Allow to cool for 10 minutes before cutting into 16 squares. Store in an airtight container at room temperature for up to 3 days.

Macros per blondie:

Calories (kCal) 165; Total Fat 10g (Saturated Fat 2g, Trans Fat 0g); Cholesterol 0mg; Sodium 60mg; Potassium 393mg; Total Carbohydrate 12g (Dietary Fiber 2g, Sugars 5g); Protein 11g

Apple-Cinnamon Protein Pudding

Makes 6 servings
Prep Time: 50 minutes, plus 1 hour chilling
Cook Time: 15 minutes

MEAL PLAN KEY: LEAN PROTEIN + HIGH CARB

If you are struggling to get more protein in your diet and can't stomach more meat, this pudding is a clever treat for the taste buds. Convenient, economical, and so good that your entire family will enjoy it, this high-protein treat is great as a make-ahead economical snack (a nice substitute for beef jerky in meal plans) or on-the-go breakfast.

Ingredients

4 cups boiling water

20 oz chopped apples (approximately 6 small apples)

2 teaspoons vanilla extract

PUDDING BASE

1 cup room-temperature water

6 scoops vanilla-flavored whey protein isolate

8 (1-gram) packets calorie-free sweetener of your choice*

2½ teaspoons xanthan gum

2 teaspoons ground cinnamon

Examples include stevia and monk fruit (aka luo han guo) sweetener.

1. Bring the 4 cups water to a boil in a medium saucepan. Add the apples and vanilla extract and bring to a boil again. Reduce the heat to medium-low and cook, uncovered and stirring occasionally, for 35 to 40 minutes, until apples are softened. Remove from heat and set aside.

2. Transfer to a food processor and add cooked apples with the 1 cup room-temperature water, the protein powder, sweetener, xanthan gum, and cinnamon. Process on high for 30 to 60 seconds, until smooth.

3. Spoon ¾ cup pudding into each of six mason jars or airtight containers and set in the fridge. Refrigerate for at least 1 hour or overnight. Keeps for up to 7 days in the fridge.

Macros per ¾-cup serving (12 tablespoons):
Calories (kCal) 165; Total Fat 0g (Saturated Fat 0g, Trans Fat 0g); Cholesterol 0mg; Sodium 92mg; Potassium 243mg; Total Carbohydrate 17g (Dietary Fiber: 4g, Sugars 10g); Protein 25g

Chocolate–Peanut Butter Zucchini Brownies

Makes 16 servings
Prep Time: 10 minutes
Cook Time: 20 minutes
MEAL PLAN KEY: FATTY LOW-GI CARB

If going low carb has you missing sweets, the search for an amazing recipe that truly satisfies your sweet tooth is over. This low-carb brownie is rich, moist, and completely decadent without adding sugar or excessive carbs. At only 5 net carbs per serving, you can easily enjoy these within your macro goals for the day!

Ingredients
Coconut oil spray
8 oz chopped zucchini
8 oz (1 cup) unsweetened almond milk
8.5 oz (1 cup) peanut butter
4.2 oz (1 cup) unsweetened cocoa powder
4 oz (4 scoops) chocolate-flavored whey protein isolate
5 (1-gram) packets calorie-free sweetener of your choice*
Examples include stevia and monk fruit (aka luo han guo) sweetener.

1. Preheat the oven to 350°F. Spray a 9 × 9-inch nonstick baking pan with coconut oil.
2. Combine all the remaining ingredients in a food processor and process on high for 1 to 2 minutes. Batter will have a smooth yet thick consistency.

3. Pour batter into the prepared pan and bake for about 20 minutes, until batter is firm.

4. Allow to cool for 10 minutes before cutting the brownies into 16 squares. Store in an airtight container at room temperature for up to 3 days (if they last that long!).

Macros per brownie:
  Calories (kCal) 139; Total Fat 10g (Saturated Fat 2g, Trans Fat 0g); Cholesterol 0mg; Sodium 102mg; Potassium 181mg; Total Carbohydrate 8g (Dietary Fiber 3g, Sugars 2g); Protein: 11g

Pumpkin Wheynola

Makes 9 servings
Prep Time: 10 minutes
Cook Time: 35 minutes

MEAL PLAN KEY: FATTY PROTEIN + LOW-GI CARB

Enjoy five times the protein with only 25 percent of the carbs found in a traditional granola recipe with amazing wheynola! You now have the ability to *add* protein to your cereal, yogurts, and smoothies and carry it around for a convenient snack when traveling. This is one of my go-to travel-friendly snacks to keep in my purse. While traveling, I can just buy a nonfat Greek yogurt and sprinkle this in for more protein and crunch. Make it more keto-friendly by eliminating the dried cranberries and chocolate chips to make more room in your day for other carbs.

Ingredients
  3.5 oz (3½ scoops) vanilla-flavored whey protein isolate
  3.1 oz (6 tablespoons) almond butter (can use Toasted Coconut–Maple Almond Butter, page 267)
  2 oz (¼ cup) water
  1 oz (4 tablespoons) pumpkin seeds
  0.2 oz (2 tablespoons) coconut chips
  0.7 oz (2 tablespoons) chocolate chips

0.5 oz (2 tablespoons) dried cranberries

2 teaspoons pumpkin pie spice

Coconut oil spray or olive oil spray

1. Preheat the oven to 300°F. Line a nonstick baking sheet with parchment paper.
2. Combine the protein powder, almond butter, water, pumpkin seeds, coconut chips, chocolate chips, dried cranberries, and pumpkin pie spice in a medium bowl to form a fudge-like texture. Spread mixture on the prepared baking sheet in an even layer.
3. Bake for 20 minutes. Using a metal spatula, break the mass apart into bite-sized pieces about the size of a quarter.
4. Lightly spray the broken pieces with oil spray and bake for 10 more minutes. Then broil for 2 to 3 minutes, watching very closely, until the wheynola is golden brown but not burnt.

Meal Prep Tips:

- Makes a great topping on Greek yogurt, a stand-alone snack, or with low-sugar fruit.
- Store in an airtight container at room temperature for 1 week.

Macros per 2-tablespoon serving (or about 1 ounce)

Calories (kCal) 161; Total Fat 9g (Saturated Fat 2g, Trans Fat 1g); Cholesterol 0mg; Sodium 62mg; Potassium 97mg; Total Carbohydrate 8g (Dietary Fiber 2g, Sugars 4g); Protein 16g

Coconut and Chocolate Chip Protein Bites

Makes 12 bites

Prep Time: 15 minutes, plus 30 minutes freezing

Cook Time: none

MEAL PLAN KEY: FATTY PROTEIN + LOW-GI CARB

My biggest pet peeve when I travel is that the majority of airports and gas stations do not have high-protein snacks that are low in fats and carbs. The average "protein bar" is loaded with carbs or too high in fat to suit my macronutrient goals. So I am left with no other option than to make my own travel-friendly protein snack. Enjoy this simple, no-bake recipe that allows the utmost in convenience while packing over 12 grams of protein per bite! Try it with your favorite flavor of protein powder.

Ingredients
  4 oz (4 scoops) vanilla-flavored whey protein isolate
  2.6 oz (5 tablespoons) almond butter (can use Toasted Coconut–
      Maple Almond Butter, page 267)
  1.4 oz (¼ cup) chocolate chunks (or chocolate chips)
  5 oz (10 tablespoons) water
  0.4 oz (2 tablespoons) shredded unsweetened coconut

1. Combine the protein powder, almond butter, and chocolate in a large bowl. Mix together using a spoon. Add the water, 1 tablespoon at a time, until the dry powder is incorporated into the nut butter. This will form a thick, firm batter. Divide into 12 (1-tablespoon) portions and roll into balls.
2. Sprinkle the shredded coconut on a small plate and roll each ball in the coconut to lightly coat.
3. Place on wax or parchment paper and set in the freezer for a minimum of 30 minutes. Store in the freezer in a plastic baggie until ready to eat.

Meal Prep Tips:
  • If frozen, best if consumed within 2 months. Can be refrigerated for 3 to 4 days.
  • Great for a convenient, high-protein, travel-friendly snack that fits inside your purse or carry-on for road trips and air travel. They are good for an afternoon or day trip.
  • Works well with a variety of protein powders.

Macros per bite/ball:
  Calories (kCal) 118; Total Fat 6g (Saturated Fat 2g, Trans Fat 0g); Cholesterol 2mg; Sodium 65mg; Potassium 217mg; Total Carbohydrate 4g (Dietary Fiber 1g, Sugars 2g); Protein 12g

High-GI Carbs (Carbs from Starches)

Spiralized Sweet Potato Fries

Makes 5 servings

Prep Time: 10 minutes

Cook Time: 30 minutes

MEAL PLAN KEY: HIGH-GI CARB

Don't settle for subpar meals just because your health is a priority. Once I realized I could spiralize sweet potatoes and transform them into crispy pieces of deliciousness, I couldn't get enough of these potato fries. It's an excellent side dish with any meal and a fun way to enjoy your complex carbohydrates. Get creative and mix it up by experimenting with other seasoning blends, like cumin or cinnamon.

Ingredients

20 oz sweet potatoes (about 2 large)

1 oz (2 tablespoons) extra-virgin olive oil

Sea salt and black pepper (to taste)

1. Preheat the oven to 400°F. Line a baking sheet with parchment paper.
2. Use a spiralizer to cut the sweet potatoes into spiralized fries. Toss the fries with the olive oil, salt, and pepper. Place on the lined baking sheet and bake for 30 minutes, or until desired level of crispness.

Macros per 4-ounce serving:

Calories (kCal) 146; Total Fat 5g (Saturated Fat 1g, Trans Fat 0g); Cholesterol 0mg; Sodium 519mg; Potassium 387mg; Total Carbohydrate 23g (Dietary Fiber 4g, Sugars 5g); Protein 2g

Garlic-Jalapeño Cilantro Rice

Makes 4 servings

Prep Time: 10 minutes, plus time to cook the rice

Cook Time: 5 minutes

MEAL PLAN KEY: HIGH-GI CARB

If you are the type of person who needs your food to be filled with flavor or you won't eat it, you'll love this recipe because it's an easy way to take a basic white rice and transform it into a savory dish. Garlic, hot peppers, and fresh herbs are all great ways to boost flavor without using additives or extra oil. The rice pairs well with chicken, fish, meat, and veggies!

Ingredients

1 oz (2 tablespoons) extra-virgin olive oil

4 cloves garlic, minced

0.5 oz (~½) jalapeño, seeded and diced

16 oz (2 cups cooked) white jasmine rice

1 oz (2 tablespoons) soy sauce*

0.14 oz (¼ cup) fresh cilantro leaves, chopped

Substitute coconut aminos for a soy-free alternative.

1. Heat the olive oil in a medium skillet over medium-high heat. Add the garlic and sauté for 30 to 45 seconds.

2. Add the jalapeño and rice and top with the soy sauce. Stir-fry for 1 minute, or until all the rice is a light brown color and the jalapeño is evenly distributed.

3. Remove from heat and top with the cilantro.

Macros per serving:

Calories (kCal) 176; Total Fat 7g (Saturated Fat 1g, Trans Fat 0g); Cholesterol 0mg; Sodium 664mg; Potassium 42 mg; Total Carbohydrate 25g (Dietary Fiber 1g, Sugars 1g); Protein 3g

Curried Coconut Rice

Makes 4 servings
Prep Time: 3 minutes, plus time to cook the rice
Cook Time: 5 minutes
MEAL PLAN KEY: HIGH-GI CARB

Keep your meal prep fresh by mixing a fun flavor profile into your rice! If you are tired of the same old foods and are in a rut, picking up a few simple spices will not only boost flavor in this easy coconut rice but will also give you something new to look forward to. If you've never had any of these ingredients before, give them a try and experience variety without adding unnecessary calories.

Ingredients
0.5 oz (1 tablespoon) coconut oil
16 oz (2 cups) cooked white jasmine rice
1 tablespoon curry powder
1 teaspoon paprika
1 teaspoon cayenne pepper
2 oz (¼ cup) unsweetened coconut milk (from a carton)
Fresh Italian parsley for garnish (optional)

1. Heat the coconut oil in a medium skillet and allow to melt for 15 to 20 seconds.
2. Add the cooked rice, curry powder, paprika, and cayenne and stir-fry for 30 seconds, or until all the rice is a light yellow color.
3. Add the coconut milk and stir-fry for another minute, until all ingredients are combined. Remove from the heat and top with parsley, if desired.

Macros per serving:
Calories (kCal) 142; Total Fat 4g (Saturated Fat 3g, Trans Fat 0g); Cholesterol 0mg; Sodium 5mg; Potassium 32mg; Total Carbohydrate 24g (Dietary Fiber 2g, Sugars 0g); Protein 2g

Mexican-Style Rice

Makes 4 servings

Prep Time: 5 minutes, plus time to cook the rice

Cook Time: 5 minutes

MEAL PLAN KEY: HIGH-GI CARB

Whether you are preparing one of the main protein dishes for an easy week-night dinner or meal prepping for the week to come, you will feel proud of yourself for this easy recipe that doesn't disappoint. Inspired by a traditional Mexican rice recipe but adapted for macro eating, this rice boasts more flavor compared to a plain white rice without the unnecessary sugars and low-quality fats from more traditional Mexican-inspired rices. Feel free to cook the rice in bulk and portion your meals off it for three or four days when you need convenience and flavor! If raw onion is too strong for your taste, sauté the onion in the coconut oil first and then stir-fry the rice.

Ingredients

0.5 oz (1 tablespoon) coconut oil

16 oz (2 cups) cooked white jasmine rice

0.43 oz (2 tablespoons) cumin

1 teaspoon paprika

Sea salt (to taste)

0.35 oz (3 tablespoons) chopped red onion

1. Heat the coconut oil in a medium skillet and allow to melt for 15 to 20 seconds.
2. Add the cooked rice, cumin, paprika, and salt and stir-fry for 30 seconds, or until all the spices are evenly distributed.
3. Remove from heat and top with chopped onion.

Macros per serving:

Calories (kCal) 157; Total Fat 4g (Saturated Fat 3g, Trans Fat 0g); Cholesterol 0mg; Sodium 7mg; Potassium 108mg; Total Carbohydrate 27g (Dietary Fiber 1g, Sugars 0g); Protein 3g

Oven-Roasted Spiced Potatoes

Makes 8 servings
Prep Time: 10 minutes
Cook Time: 35 to 40 minutes
MEAL PLAN KEY: HIGH-GI CARB

Enjoy these easy, simply seasoned roasted potatoes as an ideal side in gluten-free and grain-free breakfasts, lunches, or dinners. A high roasting temperature helps crisp the potatoes and gives them an excellent texture even after reheating! These pair well with a protein source of your choice.

Ingredients
32 oz (2 lb) tricolored potatoes, cut into ½-inch pieces
Olive oil spray
2 tablespoons paprika
2 tablespoons thyme, dried
1 tablespoon garlic powder
1 tablespoon cayenne pepper
1 tablespoon freshly ground black pepper
Sea salt (optional)
Fresh thyme sprigs for garnish (optional)

1. Preheat the oven to 400°F. Line a baking sheet with parchment paper.
2. In a small bowl, combine the paprika, thyme, garlic powder, cayenne, black pepper, and salt. In a medium mixing bowl, lightly spray the potatoes with olive oil. Add the spices and toss until they are evenly distributed. Spread out on the prepared baking sheet.
3. Roast the potatoes until almost tender, about 35 minutes. Remove from the oven and lightly spray with olive oil. Broil for 2 to 3 minutes, until lightly browned and crisped. Top with fresh sprigs of thyme if you like and toss the potatoes with tongs to evenly distribute the flavors.

Meal Prep Tips:
- Great for meal planning in bulk. Keeps for 5 days, refrigerated.
- Works well for grain-free and gluten-free breakfast skillets.

Macros per 4-ounce serving:

Calories (kCal) 171; Total Fat 7g (Saturated Fat 1g, Trans Fat 0g); Cholesterol 0mg; Sodium 789mg; Potassium 45mg; Total Carbohydrate 28g (Dietary Fiber 4g, Sugars 2g); Protein 4g

Garlic-Spinach Quinoa

Makes 4 servings

Prep Time: 5 minutes, plus time to cook the quinoa

Cook Time: 25 minutes

MEAL PLAN KEY: HIGH-GI CARB

When you want to be healthy, simple twists on basic ingredients will keep you going! This simple combination of olive oil, garlic, spinach, and a touch of soy sauce is a wonderful way to enhance the flavor of quinoa.

Ingredients

1 tablespoon extra-virgin olive oil

2 cloves garlic, minced

2 oz (2 cups) spinach, chopped

16 oz (2 cups) cooked quinoa

1 oz (2 tablespoons) low-sodium soy sauce*

Substitute coconut aminos for a soy-free alternative.

1. Heat the olive oil in a skillet over medium-high heat. Add the garlic and sauté for 30 to 45 seconds.

2. Add the spinach and cook down for 30 seconds, until just wilted.

3. Add the cooked quinoa and soy sauce and stir-fry for 2 minutes, until flavors are evenly distributed.

Macros per ½-cup serving:

Calories (kCal) 157; Total Fat 5g (Saturated Fat 1g, Trans Fat 0g); Cholesterol 0mg; Sodium 249mg; Potassium 249mg; Total Carbohydrate 22g (Dietary Fiber 3g, Sugars 1g); Protein 6g

Cumin-Cilantro Sweet Potatoes

Makes 5 servings
Prep Time: 10 minutes
Total Cook Time: 45 minutes
MEAL PLAN KEY: HIGH-GI CARB

I love the convenience and natural sweetness of sweet potatoes. Not only are they a low-cost carb source, but they are easy to prepare in bulk and are an amazing source of vitamin A in the form of beta carotene. They are also a good source of fiber and are excellent with this savory blend of spices.

Ingredients
Olive oil spray
20 oz sweet potatoes, rinsed and cut into ¼-inch slices
0.3 oz (3 tablespoons) fresh chopped cilantro
0.43 oz (2 tablespoons) ground cumin
1 teaspoon garlic powder
¼ teaspoon cayenne pepper
Sea salt and black pepper (to taste)

1. Preheat the oven to 350°F. Line a baking sheet with foil and lightly spray with olive oil.
2. In a small bowl, combine the cilantro, cumin, garlic powder, cayenne, salt, and pepper. Place the sweet potatoes on the baking sheet and lightly spray with olive oil. Sprinkle with the spices and toss well.
3. Arrange the potatoes in one layer and roast, tossing occasionally, for 30 minutes, until the potatoes are tender and golden brown. Broil for 3 to 5 minutes for extra-crispy potatoes, watching carefully to ensure they don't burn. Let cool for 5 to 10 minutes before serving.

Macros per 4-ounce serving:
Calories (kCal) 114; Total Fat 1g (Saturated Fat 0g, Trans Fat 0g); Cholesterol 0mg; Sodium 520mg; Potassium 436mg; Total Carbohydrate 24g (Dietary Fiber 4g, Sugars 5g); Protein 2g

Low-GI Carbs (Carbs from Veggies)

Oven-Roasted Eggplant and Bell Pepper Medley

Makes 4 servings
Prep Time: 15 minutes
Cook Time: 45 minutes
MEAL PLAN KEY: LOW-GI CARB

My most successful clients are the ones who are the most open-minded about exploring new ingredients. Learning new ways to get nutrients with foods you enjoy is key to a sustainable healthy lifestyle. Try this fun medley of eggplant, bell pepper, and fresh basil for an all-natural way to hit your fiber content!

Ingredients
  24 oz eggplant (about 2 medium)
  Sea salt and black pepper
  Olive oil spray
  5 cloves garlic, minced
  0.2 oz (2 tablespoons) dried oregano
  12 oz (~3 tricolor bell peppers), cored, seeded, and chopped
  0.12 oz (3 tablespoons) fresh chopped basil

1. Preheat the oven to 350°F and line a baking sheet with parchment paper.
2. Trim the ends from the eggplants. Cut each in half lengthwise and then in half again. Slice each quarter into four pieces. Place on paper towels and liberally rub with sea salt. Let the eggplant sweat out excess moisture for 10 minutes.
3. Dab the eggplant "sweat" with paper towels and rub off the salt. Place the eggplant on the prepared baking sheet and spray with olive oil. Top evenly with the garlic, oregano, and salt and pepper to taste. Roast for 30 minutes.

4. Remove from the oven and add the bell peppers. Season with salt and pepper and spray with olive oil. Return to the oven and roast for 15 to 20 minutes, until the eggplant has a soft creamy texture and the peppers are softened. Finish by broiling for 1 minute to crisp. Let cool for 10 minutes before topping with the chopped basil.

Macros per serving:

Calories (kCal) 66; Total Fat 1g (Saturated Fat 0g, Trans Fat 0g); Cholesterol 1mg; Sodium 595mg; Potassium 434mg; Total Carbohydrate 14g (Dietary Fiber 7g, Sugars 6g); Protein 2g

Lemon-Garlic Kale Sauté

Makes 4 servings
Prep Time: 5 minutes
Cook Time: 2 minutes
MEAL PLAN KEY: LOW-GI CARB

This savory kale dish is nutrient-dense and vegan-friendly. It will help maintain high levels of iron to keep your energy level up, with an added bonus of vitamin C from the lemon. This superfood side dish comes together in just a few minutes, pairs well with any main dish, and does not disappoint.

Ingredients

Olive oil spray
2 cloves garlic, minced
4 cups chopped kale
Juice from 1 lemon
Sea salt and black pepper (to taste)

1. Lightly spray a large skillet with olive oil. Add garlic and sauté over medium heat for 30 to 45 seconds until lightly golden. Add the kale and cook over medium-high heat for 1 minute, until kale is slightly wilted.
2. Pour the lemon juice over the kale and stir-fry for 1 minute, until cooked down and flavor is evenly distributed. Season with salt and pepper to taste.

Meal Prep Tips:

- Batch cooking and reheating are not recommended, as reheated veggies tend to be soggy.
- Keep a large bag of leafy greens on hand, prep all other elements of your meal, and sauté the greens either right before you eat or that morning if possible.

Macros per serving:

Calories (kCal) 36; Total Fat 0g (Saturated Fat 0g, Trans Fat 0g); Cholesterol 0mg; Sodium 599mg; Potassium 335mg; Total Carbohydrate 7g (Dietary Fiber 1g, Sugars 0g); Protein 2g

Garlic-Veggie Lentil Salad

Makes 4 servings

Prep Time: 10 minutes, plus time to cook the lentils

Cook Time: 5 minutes

MEAL PLAN KEY: LOW-GI CARB

Lentils are one of the most underrated plant-based protein sources. They are high in protein, full of fiber, vegan-friendly, and are so good that even meat lovers will be pleasantly surprised by their ability to adapt to a wide variety of flavors. This recipe is a great hit if you want to mix it up, if you are pursuing more plant-based protein sources in your diet, or if you need to prepare a vegan-friendly dish for guests.

Ingredients

1 tablespoon extra-virgin olive oil

3 cloves garlic, minced

4 oz (1 medium) red bell pepper, cored, seeded, and chopped

1 oz carrot (½ medium) carrot, chopped

5.3 oz (2 cups) cooked lentils

6 oz (½ cup) frozen peas

Sea salt and black pepper (to taste)

Squeeze of lemon (optional)

1. Heat the olive oil in a medium nonstick skillet over medium-high heat. Add the garlic and sauté for 30 to 60 seconds.
2. Add the bell pepper and carrot and stir-fry for another 60 seconds. Reduce the heat to medium and add the lentils and peas. Stir-fry for another minute, until all veggies are mixed yet still bright and crisp and not too soft.
3. Remove from the heat and let cool for 5 to 10 minutes before serving with a squeeze of lemon. Season with salt and black pepper to taste.

Macros per 4-ounce serving:
Calories (kCal) 188; Total Fat 4g (Saturated Fat 1g, Trans Fat 0g); Cholesterol 0mg; Sodium 651mg; Potassium 555mg; Total Carbohydrate 28g (Dietary Fiber 11g, Sugars 5g); Protein 11g

Asparagus Sauté

Makes 4 servings
Prep Time: 5 minutes
Cook Time: 8 minutes
MEAL PLAN KEY: LOW-GI CARB

Get inspired by asparagus again with this fresh take on the tried-and-true healthy ingredient. The light and savory sauté is rich in flavor, with only 1 gram of net carbs for the win!

Ingredients
16 oz (1 lb) thin asparagus, tough ends trimmed
3 slices bacon
2 cloves garlic, minced
6 Kalamata olives, sliced
1 teaspoon red pepper flakes
¼ teaspoon sea salt

1. Cut the asparagus stalks at a 45-degree angle into 2-inch pieces.
2. Cook the bacon in a medium skillet over medium-high heat until crisp; set the bacon aside, reserving the grease in the pan.

3. Add the garlic to the bacon grease and sauté over medium-high heat for 30 to 45 seconds. Add the asparagus and olives and stir-fry for 3 to 4 minutes, until the asparagus is softened but still a bright green color.

4. Crumble or chop the bacon into small pieces. Transfer the asparagus to a serving bowl, top with the crumbled bacon, and season with red pepper flakes and salt.

Macros per ½-cup serving:
Calories (kCal) 69; Total Fat 4g (Saturated Fat 1g, Trans Fat 0g); Cholesterol 6mg; Sodium 633mg; Potassium 81mg; Total Carbohydrate 5g (Dietary Fiber 4g, Sugars 4g); Protein 6g

Roasted Brussels Sprouts and Purple Cauliflower

Makes 8 servings
Prep Time: 5 minutes
Cook Time: 40 minutes
MEAL PLAN KEY: LOW-GI CARB

Add some color to your plate with a simple, nutrient-dense dish of oven-roasted veggies. Purple cauliflower is a seasonal vegetable whose vibrant color comes from anthocyanin, an antioxidant also found in red wine. Enjoy this simple side dish of superfoods to balance out any main dish.

Ingredients
16 oz (about 1 lb) purple cauliflower (1 medium head), stemmed and cut into florets
16 oz (1 lb) Brussels sprouts, stemmed and halved
1 oz (2 tablespoons) extra-virgin olive oil
1 teaspoon black pepper
¼ teaspoon sea salt

1. Preheat the oven to 400°F. Line a baking sheet with parchment paper.
2. Toss the cauliflower and Brussels sprouts in a medium bowl with the olive oil, pepper, and salt.

3. Arrange the veggies on the baking sheet with the sprouts cut-side down so that the leaves can crisp. Roast for 40 minutes, until lightly crisped.

Macro per ½-cup serving:

Calories (kCal) 70; Total Fat 4g (Saturated Fat 1g, Trans Fat 0g); Cholesterol 0mg; Sodium 251mg; Potassium 224mg; Total Carbohydrate 8g (Dietary Fiber 3g, Sugars 2g); Protein 3g

Rosemary-Roasted Butternut Squash

Makes 8 servings
Prep Time: 10 minutes
Cook Time: 30 minutes
MEAL PLAN KEY: LOW-GI CARB

If you are unable to digest gluten, butternut squash is a great alternative to gluten-based carbs like oats, bread, pasta, etc. I fell in love with this winter squash not only because it tastes great but because it is very low in carbohydrates yet leaves you feeling completely full and satisfied. This is an incredible dish on its own, but it pairs well with chicken, lentils, or the protein source of your choice.

Ingredients

Olive oil spray

32 oz (about 2 lb) butternut squash (1 large), peeled, seeded, and cut into 1-inch chunks

2 sprigs fresh rosemary

Sea salt and black pepper (to taste)

1. Preheat the oven to 400°F. Line a baking sheet with foil and lightly spray with olive oil.
2. Place the squash on the baking sheet and lightly spray with olive oil, then add the rosemary, salt, and pepper and toss. Arrange the squash in one layer and roast, stirring occasionally, for 30 minutes, until the squash is tender and golden brown.

Macros per 4-ounce serving:

> Calories (kCal) 55; Total Fat 0g (Saturated Fat 0g, Trans Fat 0g); Cholesterol 0mg; Sodium 291mg; Potassium 4mg; Total Carbohydrate 13g (Dietary Fiber 3g, Sugars 2g); Protein 1g

Lemon-Parmesan Roasted Brussels Sprouts

Makes 4 servings

Prep Time: 10 minutes

Cook Time: 35 minutes

MEAL PLAN KEY: LOW-GI CARB

If you have written off Brussels sprouts, this recipe will have you reconsidering everything you thought you knew about the cruciferous veggie. Peeling apart the sprouts allows them to get crispy and delicious. With a crust of Parmesan and a touch of lemon, it's an incredible side dish for the entrée of your choice and a nice touch at holiday gatherings.

Ingredients

> Olive oil spray
>
> 16 oz Brussels sprouts, stemmed and quartered
>
> 1 oz lemon juice (~juice of 1 lemon)
>
> 1.6 oz (½ cup) grated Parmesan cheese
>
> Sea salt and black pepper (to taste)

1. Preheat the oven to 350°F. Line a baking sheet tray with foil and lightly spray with olive oil.
2. Carefully peel apart the outer leaves of the prepped sprouts and break them down to allow for a more leaf-like texture as opposed to a solid sprout.
3. Arrange the Brussels sprouts on the baking sheet in one layer. Toss with the lemon juice and sprinkle with the Parmesan cheese. Roast for 30 minutes, until tender and the tips of the leaves are a golden brown. Broil for 3 to 5 minutes for an extra-crispy finish, but watch carefully to ensure the sprouts do not burn.

4. Let cool for 5 to 10 minutes, season with salt and pepper to taste, and serve.

Macros per 4-ounce serving:
Calories (kCal) 98; Total Fat 4g (Saturated Fat 2g, Trans Fat 0g); Cholesterol 7mg; Sodium 774mg; Potassium 16mg; Total Carbohydrate 9g (Dietary Fiber 4g, Sugars 3g); Protein 6g

Spicy Garlic Dill Pickles

Makes 14 servings
Prep Time: 10 minutes
Cook Time: none
MEAL PLAN KEY: COUNTLESS FOOD

Anyone who has been a part of my private online community knows that pickles are a free (countless) food. This means you can eat them freely on your program without having to count the calories because they are so low. If you have a pang for salty foods, this is a great way to curb cravings! If you can't obtain Filipino spiced vinegar, add hot dried chile peppers to white vinegar for a similar effect.

Ingredients
12 oz (1½ cups) Filipino spiced vinegar
0.15 oz (½ cup) coarsely chopped fresh dill
3 cloves garlic, minced
4 teaspoons sea salt
1 teaspoon red pepper
4 oz (½ cup) boiling water
14 oz Persian cucumbers (about 6), cut lengthwise into ¼-inch slices

1. Combine the vinegar, dill, garlic, salt, and pepper in a 1-quart mason jar, cover, and shake well.
2. Add the boiling water and make sure that the salt dissolves.
3. Add the cucumbers to the jar, cover, and refrigerate overnight. The pickles will keep in the fridge for 30 days.

Macros per 1-ounce serving:
  Calories (kCal) 20; Total Fat 0g (Saturated Fat 0g, Trans Fat 0g); Cholesterol 0mg; Sodium 690mg; Potassium 85mg; Total Carbohydrate 2g (Dietary Fiber 1g, Sugars 1g); Protein 0g

Shishito Peppers

Makes 8 servings
Prep Time: 25 minutes
Cook Time: 30 minutes
MEAL PLAN KEY: COUNTLESS FOOD

The first time I tried shishito peppers, I was in New York City at a business dinner. I was blown away by this seemingly light appetizer that was mild tasting with a touch of char and sea salt. Once back home, I re-created it, but with less fat and a squeeze of lemon, and finished it with black truffle sea salt to take the peppers to the next level. Serve as a healthy appetizer or side to any meal.

Ingredients
  8 oz whole shishito peppers
  Olive oil spray
  Squeeze of lemon (optional)
  Black truffle sea salt (optional)

1. Place the peppers in a nonstick skillet and spray with olive oil. Turn the heat to high and let the oiled peppers sit for 30 to 60 seconds, then stir-fry for 1 to 2 minutes, allowing them to char but watching closely so they don't burn. Reduce the heat to medium-high and continue to cook the peppers until they are slightly wilted, softened, and blistered (popping is normal — this blistering adds a unique texture). This should take 6 to 8 minutes.
2. Let sit for a minute, then transfer to a plate or bowl and top with a squeeze of lemon and a generous sprinkling of truffle sea salt if you like.

Macros per 2-ounce serving:

Calories (kCal) 35; Total Fat 2.3g (Saturated Fat 8g, Trans Fat 0g); Cholesterol 0mg; Sodium 152mg; Total Carbohydrate 2.7g (Dietary Fiber 0.7g, Sugars 2g); Protein 1.3g

Filipino Eggplant Adobo

Makes 10 servings

Prep Time: 15 minutes

Cook Time: 25 minutes

MEAL PLAN KEY: LOW-GI CARB

Adobo is a popular Filipino dish of chicken or pork cooked in vinegar, soy sauce, garlic, bay leaves, and black pepper. I was inspired to prepare eggplant in this amazing sauce after a trip to Philadelphia's Chinatown, where I found the prettiest bright-purple Chinese eggplants that needed a special preparation.

Ingredients

6 Chinese eggplants (about 45 oz)

Sea salt

Olive oil spray

2 oz (¼ cup) extra-virgin olive oil

2 oz (¼ cup) coarsely chopped garlic

4 bay leaves

4 oz (½ cup) soy sauce*

2 oz (¼ cup) vinegar of your choice

1 teaspoon freshly ground black pepper

3 oz (⅓ cup) water

2 oz (2 cups) spinach

Use coconut aminos for a soy-free alternative.

1. Trim the tops and bottoms from the eggplants, then slice in half lengthwise. Cut into approximately 1½-inch pieces. Sprinkle salt over the eggplant and let sit for 5 to 10 minutes to sweat out the water. Press on the

tops with paper towels to absorb the water. Pat a few times and then brush off the excess salt.

2. Lightly spray a nonstick wok with olive oil. Add the ¼ cup olive oil, garlic, and bay leaves and lightly sauté over high heat for 30 to 45 seconds.

3. Add all the eggplant to the wok and stir-fry for about 1 minute. Add the soy sauce, vinegar, black pepper, and water and continue to stir-fry for 15 to 20 minutes to cook down the eggplant and concentrate the sauce until the eggplant is softened.

4. Add the spinach and cook down for about 1 minute and then remove from heat.

Macros per serving:
Calories (kCal) 101; Total Fat 6g (Saturated Fat 1g, Trans Fat 0g); Cholesterol 0mg; Sodium 1,062mg; Potassium 50mg; Total Carbohydrate 12g (Dietary Fiber 5g, Sugars 5g); Protein 3g

Healthy Fats

Garlic-Rosemary Butter

Makes 16 servings
Prep Time: 5 minutes
Cook Time: 15 minutes
MEAL PLAN KEY: HEALTHY FAT

Take your butter to the next level with this mind-blowing, naturally flavored source of healthy fats. This flavored butter is an excellent way to cook veggies and meat, or use as a topping.

Ingredients
5 cloves garlic, peeled
2 sticks (8 oz) salted grass-fed butter
2 sprigs fresh rosemary

Juice of ½ lemon

¼ teaspoon sea salt

½ teaspoon black pepper

1. Roast the garlic: Preheat the oven to 350°F. Wrap the garlic cloves in one piece of foil. Place directly on the oven rack and roast for 15 to 20 minutes and then set aside.
2. In a medium bowl, microwave the butter at 80 percent power for 30 seconds, until softened.
3. Add the roasted garlic, rosemary, lemon juice, salt, and pepper to the butter and mix with a handheld immersion blender for a few pulses, until combined.
4. Refrigerate in an airtight container.

Meal Prep Tips:

- Great to prepare ahead if you are on lower-carb and higher-fat macros as an easy way to boost fat content and add flavor to proteins like steak, chicken, and seafood
- Keeps in the fridge for 7 to 10 days.

Macros per 1 tablespoon:
Calories (kCal) 104; Total Fat 12g (Saturated Fat 7g, Trans Fat 0g); Cholesterol 31mg; Sodium 230mg; Potassium 10mg; Total Carbohydrate 0g (Dietary Fiber 0g, Sugars 0g); Protein 0g

Pesto

Makes 7 servings
Prep Time: 10 minutes, plus time to roast the garlic
Cook Time: none
MEAL PLAN KEY: HEALTHY FAT

I am obsessed with the rich flavor of simple ingredients like basil, garlic, and olive oil. There is zero comparison between this fresh basil sauce made from real whole foods and store-bought pesto. My fragrant pesto is an incredible addition to pasta dishes, veggies, salmon, chicken, meatballs, and much more. Make it when you want a break from dairy- or tomato-based sauces.

Ingredients

0.6 oz (6 cloves) roasted garlic (see Garlic-Rosemary Butter, page 263)

0.7 oz (1 cup) coarsely chopped fresh basil

0.25 oz (¼ cup) chopped spinach

4 oz (½ cup) extra-virgin olive oil

0.5 oz lemon juice (juice of ½ lemon)

0.5 oz sundried tomato (optional)

1 teaspoon oregano

1 teaspoon sea salt

¼ teaspoon black pepper

1. Combine all the ingredients in a food processor and pulse for 15 to 20 seconds until emulsified.
2. Store in an airtight container in the fridge for up to 3 to 4 days.

Macros per serving (about 1 tablespoon):
Calories (kCal) 146; Total Fat 16g (Saturated Fat 2g, Trans Fat 0g); Cholesterol 0mg; Sodium 341mg; Potassium 73mg; Total Carbohydrate 2g (Dietary Fiber 0g, Sugars 0g); Protein 1g

Hot Chili Oil

Makes 48 servings
Prep Time: 10 minutes
Cook Time: 60 minutes
MEAL PLAN KEY: HEALTHY FAT

Meet your new favorite condiment! Growing up, I used to get Chinese food with my mom at the mall every week on her pay day. She always asked for hot chili oil on the side, and I became hooked on the rich spicy flavor from a young age. One day I finally tried to re-create it, and to my shock and amazement, I had no idea that the complexity of the flavor was so much more than just oil and hot peppers. This sauce is special to me and something I use to this day to season simple meals like steamed chicken and mixed vegetables. Get ready to experience an insane, quality flavor with this homemade chili oil.

Ingredients

8 oz (1 cup) extra-virgin olive oil
0.4 oz (4 cloves) chopped garlic
0.33 oz (¼ cup) dried bird's beak chile peppers, chopped (leave seeds)
5 star anise pods
4 bay leaves
2 cinnamon sticks
1 teaspoon chili powder
Sea salt (to taste)
Fresh ginger (optional)

1. Heat the oil in a small skillet over medium-high heat. Add the garlic, sauté for 30 seconds, and reduce the heat to low. Add the chile peppers, anise, bay leaves, cinnamon, and chili powder. Bring to a low simmer and simmer, stirring occasionally, for an hour, until oil has turned a deep reddish-brown hue.

2. Store finished oil in a glass jar at room temperature for 2 to 3 months. It will keep for 6 months if stored in the fridge. You can strain the oil and discard the solid ingredients if desired (I personally enjoy them). Add sea salt to taste (optional). Try with ginger as a variation.

Macros per 1-teaspoon serving:

Calories (kCal) 36; Total Fat 4g (Saturated Fat 0g, Trans Fat 0g); Cholesterol 0g; Sodium 19mg (without adding salt); Potassium 7mg; Total Carbohydrate 0.4g (Dietary Fiber 0g, Sugars 0g); Protein 0g

Toasted Coconut–Maple Almond Butter

Makes about 35 servings
Prep Time: 30 minutes
Cook Time: 6 minutes
MEAL PLAN KEY: HEALTHY FAT

This recipe takes a patient person, but the result is entirely worth the wait. I have always been a fan of almond butter, but after I tasted the insanely rich, clean, and natural flavor of a nut butter that was ground before my very eyes, I was hooked. You will never want to purchase your nut butter again after you realize how much better it can be when you make it yourself from real ingredients with zero additives! Just be sure to use a high-quality food processor, as the butter requires substantial processing time.

Ingredients
   6 oz (2 cups) raw coconut chips
   9.2 oz (2 cups) raw almonds
   2 tablespoons maple syrup
   1 tablespoon coconut butter
   1 teaspoon vanilla extract
   ¼ teaspoon sea salt

1. Preheat the oven to 350°F and line a baking sheet with parchment paper. Spread the coconut chips on the baking sheet and bake for 6 minutes, until chips are lightly browned.
2. Transfer the coconut to a food processor and add the remaining ingredients. Pulse together for a few seconds, until the ingredients begin to form a crumbly consistency. Allow the food processor to run for 5 to 10 minutes. Carefully watch to ensure that your processor does not overheat, and pause every 30 to 60 seconds or so to redistribute contents from accumulating on the processor walls. Repeat the process of pausing and redistributing the contents three or four times, until a butter-like consistency is formed. This will require patience but is worth the wait.

3. Store in an airtight container at room temperature for up to 3 months
   until ready to use. Store in the fridge after opening.

Macros per 1-tablespoon serving:
    Calories (kCal) 100; Total Fat 9g (Saturated Fat 4g, Trans Fat 0g); Cholesterol 0mg;
    Sodium 71mg; Potassium 3mg; Total Carbohydrate 4g (Dietary Fiber 1g, Sugars 1g);
    Protein 2g

Chimichurri

Makes 9 servings
Prep Time: 10 minutes
Cook Time: none
MEAL PLAN KEY: HEALTHY FAT

This South American condiment, originally paired with steak in Argentina,
is typically heavier in oil, but this lightened version keeps it healthy for pairing with the meat or veggies of your choice. Enjoy as a tangy herbal sauce or
as a marinade for grilling your favorite cut of steak.

Ingredients
    0.84 oz (1½ cups) chopped fresh cilantro
    0.5 oz (½ cup) chopped fresh Italian parsley
    0.6 oz (6 cloves) garlic, peeled
    1.5 oz (3 tablespoons) lime juice
    1 oz (2 tablespoons) apple cider vinegar
    1 oz (2 tablespoons) extra-virgin olive oil
    1 teaspoon cumin
    ½ teaspoon red pepper flakes
    ½ teaspoon black pepper
    ¼ teaspoon sea salt

1. Combine all the ingredients in a food processor and pulse for 15 to
   20 seconds until liquefied.
2. Store in an airtight container in the refrigerator for up to 3 or 4 days.

Macros per 1-tablespoon serving:
    Calories (kCal) 35; Total Fat 3g (Saturated Fat 0g, Trans Fat 0g); Cholesterol 0mg;
    Sodium 269mg; Potassium 37mg; Total Carbohydrate 2g (Dietary Fiber 0g, Sugars 0g);
    Protein 0g

One-Ingredient Coconut Butter

Makes about 10 servings
Prep Time: 15 minutes
Cook Time: none
MEAL PLAN KEY: HEALTHY FAT

My biggest pet peeve with coconut oils is that the fiber has been removed. If you are on a low-carb or keto protocol, know that you can easily make your own high-quality coconut butter to help you hit your fiber goals. This simple recipe only requires one ingredient, but make sure you use a quality food processor or high-powered blender.

Ingredients
    6.4 oz (3 cups) organic unsweetened coconut chips

1. In a food processor or high-powered blender, process coconut on high for 10 to 15 minutes until liquefied. Pause every 30 to 60 seconds to wipe down sides and redistribute the coconut back to the blades to prevent overheating.
2. If the coconut will not liquefy, you can add a small amount of coconut oil to accelerate the process.
3. Store in an airtight container at room temperature for up to 30 days.

Macros per 1-tablespoon serving:
    Calories (kCal) 115; Total Fat 10g (Saturated Fat 9g, Trans Fat 0g); Cholesterol 0mg;
    Sodium 5mg; Potassium 0mg; Total Carbohydrate 4g (Dietary Fiber 2g, Sugars 1g);
    Protein 1g

Simple Mayo

Makes 9 servings

Prep Time: 5 minutes

Cook Time: none

MEAL PLAN KEY: HEALTHY FAT

You can enjoy a high-quality mayo without unnecessary additives using this fail-proof recipe. It uses staple ingredients for a smooth and light, healthy fat source that pairs well with lean protein.

Ingredients

3 large egg yolks*

3.4 oz (¾ cup) extra-virgin olive oil

0.5 oz lemon juice (juice of ½ lemon)

1 teaspoon apple cider vinegar

¼ teaspoon paprika

¼ teaspoon garlic powder

¼ teaspoon dry mustard powder (or Dijon mustard)

* Consumption of raw or undercooked eggs may increase the risk of foodborne illness.

1. Combine all the ingredients in a food processor and pulse for 15 to 20 seconds.
2. Store in an airtight container in the refrigerator for up to 14 days.

Macros per 1-tablespoon serving:

Calories (kCal) 180; Total Fat 20g (Saturated Fat 3g, Trans Fat 0g); Cholesterol 0mg; Sodium 1mg; Potassium 7mg; Total Carbohydrate 0g (Dietary Fiber 0g, Sugars 0g); Protein 1g

Keto Everything Sauce

Makes 16 servings

Prep Time: 10 minutes, plus 20 minutes in refrigerator

Cook Time: none

MEAL PLAN KEY: HEALTHY FAT

If you've been looking for a carb-free replacement for a "goes with every-thing" condiment, the search is over. This secret sauce not only tastes in-credible, but it is also easy to make and goes well with everything from meat, veggies, eggs, to . . . just about anything that needs a kick of flavor. Your friends and family will be asking you for this recipe!

Ingredients
   0.84 oz (1½ cups) chopped fresh cilantro
   4 oz (1 cup) shredded cheddar cheese
   4 oz fresh jalapeños (~4), coarsely chopped (seeds optional)
   1 clove garlic, minced
   1 large egg yolk*
   3.4 oz (¾ cup) extra-virgin olive oil
   1 oz lime juice
   1 oz lemon juice
   2 teaspoons apple cider vinegar
   1 teaspoon paprika
   ¼ teaspoon cayenne pepper
   ¼ teaspoon xanthan gum
   Consumption of raw or undercooked eggs may increase the risk of foodborne illness.

1. Combine all ingredients in a food processor and process for 2 to 3 minutes.
2. Pour contents into a mason jar or airtight storage container and refrigerate 20 minutes minimum or overnight. Keeps in the fridge for 2 weeks.

Macros per 1-tablespoon serving:
   Calories (kCal) 139; Total Fat 13g (Saturated Fat 3g, Trans Fat 0g); Cholesterol 20mg; Sodium 99mg; Potassium 155mg; Total Carbohydrate 3g (Dietary Fiber 2g, Sugars 2g); Protein 3g

9

Exercising for Your Macro Type

I never planned for a career in fitness; I just wanted abs like Janet Jackson. Little did I know that my quest for abs would change my entire life and the lives of tens of thousands of women and men all over the world.

As a nutrition and health expert, influencer, and athlete, the key to my success has always been in setting short- and long-term goals. The first step toward achieving any goal is to take your vision of what you want to achieve and build an actionable plan around it that you can follow week after week. **Failure to plan is planning to fail.** If you have been winging it with your training, it's time to take it up a notch with more intention. Sure, some activity is better than none, but if you are going to put in the effort, I say let's approach it with more strategy.

If you are reading this book, you most likely have a sincere desire to do things the *right* way. You acknowledge that shortcuts do not last. You also know that if you don't start to feel and see changes in the first few weeks, you will get discouraged quickly. My training methods are practical, to-the-point, and geared more toward aesthetic goals, not athletic performance. Yes, you will improve your strength and stamina using my methods, but fat loss happens in the kitchen, and a firm and shapely physique is built through resistance training.

YOUR FITNESS GLOSSARY

If you're new to lifting weights, I've created this helpful list of terms you will need to know, as many of these words and phrases are slang used by those who are more familiar with the gym life.

REPS: This is an abbreviated form of *repetitions,* which is the number of times a specific movement is repeated. For example, if you are doing squats, each time you squat down and stand back up is considered 1 rep.

SETS: A set is a series or group of reps. If a workout calls for 3 × 15 bicep curls, this means 3 sets of 15 reps. You do 15 reps (1 set) of bicep curls and then rest. You then do 2 more sets of 15 reps until 3 sets have been completed.

REST BETWEEN SETS: This is the amount of time you allow your muscles to recuperate between sets. For example, if you are doing 3 × 15 bicep curls, the rest between sets is the amount of time you wait before doing the next set. Perform 15 reps of bicep curls, then rest for the suggested time interval. Then do the second set of 15 reps, and then rest again for the suggested time interval. This cycle is repeated until the number of sets has been completed. It's important to optimize the rest time between sets for your macro type so they are long enough for the muscles to recover but not so long that they get cold and are no longer warmed up and activated.

SUPERSET: This is typically used as a verb, for instance "supersetting two exercises." It means you go back and forth between two exercises with zero rest between sets. The "rest" is substituted with doing the next exercise. For example, let's say you are doing 3 sets of two different exercises. You start by doing 10 reps of bench press, but instead of resting between sets, you move on to triceps extensions, then go back to bench press. Repeat this pattern, going back and forth until you complete all 6 sets. The key is to make sure that the exercises in your superset are working two different muscle groups so that, even though you aren't resting between sets, the muscle group you just worked is getting a break. The benefit of supersetting two movements is to reduce your training time as well as to boost calories burned.

TRAINING VOLUME: The term *training volume* is often used in the bodybuilding community to describe the amount of work you are doing with respect to lifting weights. This is defined as the total number of pounds lifted for a given exercise. For example, if you are squatting 100 pounds for 5 repetitions, your training volume is 100 pounds × 5 reps = 500 pounds, where if you increased your number of reps from 5 to 10 at the same amount of weight, you just doubled your training volume.

FAILURE: The term *failure* (or *muscular failure*) means to perform a given exercise until you can no longer execute the given movement with proper form. This means that your muscles have "failed" in the sense that they are exhausted. When performing a given exercise "to failure," the number of reps isn't necessarily assigned. This means that you will be performing a much higher number of reps until your muscles "fail" and you can't possibly do another movement. Failure in this case is a success, as it signals the muscle to grow so it doesn't fail next time you reach that same training volume.

AMRAP: This acronym stands for "as many reps as possible," which is typically synonymous with the term *failure* (above).

1RM: This stands for "1 rep max." It's the maximum weight you could lift with good form for 1 single repetition of a given exercise. This is a valuable piece of information to have when determining how much weight to lift for your working sets. For instance, it may be suggested to lift at 60 percent of your 1RM; so if your 1RM for a barbell squat is 100 pounds, then your working weight for the set would be 60 pounds.

COMPOUND MOVEMENT: An exercise that works more than one muscle group is a *compound movement*. Examples include deadlifts, pull-ups, shoulder presses, and kettlebell swings. These movements are beneficial due to their ability to work multiple muscles at the same time, allowing you to train more effectively in less time.

ISOLATION MOVEMENT: An exercise that works a single joint or muscle is an *isolation movement*. Examples include bicep curls, leg curls, and triceps extensions. These movements are beneficial for aesthetic purposes, where exercise results in larger muscles but not necessarily stronger muscles.

PLYOMETRICS: These exercises are explosive movements known for their ability to boost power and speed. They also burn a lot of calories. The most common examples include jumping movements, a variety of explosive push-ups, and medicine ball movements.

It's important to work out using a method that best serves your specific needs. Your ideal training volume will depend on your macro type. Some macro types experience better results using lower weight and higher reps, and others experience the complete opposite. However, a lean muscular aesthetic is not only a function of training volume alone. Far too often I see people simply go through the motions with their workouts and then wonder why they aren't getting the results they want. The key is to make sure you perform each set in a way that is actually challenging. This is the only way to stimulate muscle growth. To train effectively, be sure to move the weight through the full range of motion of the exercise. Ever see someone on the leg press with almost every plate on the rack, and they only lower it a few inches? Don't be *that* guy or gal who tries to do too much weight and sacrifices form and range of motion. Perform each movement properly by going deep enough to stimulate muscle growth. Before we get into training specifics for each macro type, it's important for all types to know how to properly select an appropriate weight to support progressive overload and to use the correct range of motion for *hypertrophy* (muscle growth).

SELECT AN APPROPRIATE WEIGHT. When you begin a new weight-training regime, start the first set of a given exercise with a modest weight. This way, you can ensure that you're able to perform the exercise properly, and you'll know how it feels to engage the muscles without injury. Once you get the basic form down, to see real progress, the weight needs to be heavy enough to challenge you to the point that by the last 1 to 2 reps, your muscles are burning and you feel as if you can't do any more (muscular failure).

INCREASE TRAINING VOLUME AS YOU GO. If you lift the same weight over and over, workout after workout, and never challenge yourself to lift heavier or perform more reps, your ability to grow fat-burning muscle will be significantly compromised. Keep in mind that you won't be able to go up in weight with every lift in every single exercise for every workout, so be sure to record your progress and take notes. Last but not least, be careful not to risk injuring yourself by lifting too heavy too soon. You won't experience any gains if you are injured.

USE THE CORRECT REP RANGE FOR HYPERTROPHY. *Muscular hypertrophy* is the technical term that describes the growth of muscle cells in size and number. In order for this to occur, you need to perform a certain number of reps at a high enough weight to signal the muscle that it must rise to the challenge and grow. A general rule of thumb for effective muscle growth is a rep range of 6 to 15 reps per exercise. This number varies based on your macro type, so be sure to pay attention to the optimal range for you. As you know by now, two individuals with two different macro types doing the same exact workouts *cannot* expect the same results. This is because the main factors that impact how well your body will respond to a given training method depend on certain parameters related to macro types.

Here are three key areas where your macro type affects your training:

1. Your Ability to Build Muscle

Some individuals, namely Fat-Fueled Macro Types, naturally have a fuller, more muscular build, while Carb-Fueled Macro Types are what bodybuilders call *hard gainers,* as they seriously struggle to add size. The protein-fueled types fall somewhere in between. If you struggle to add muscle mass, you can optimize your efforts by dialing in the correct volume of challenging sets for the targeted muscle group you wish to develop. The correct values for your goals will be provided in your macro type's detailed workout plan.

2. How Effectively Your Body Utilizes Fat for Fuel

Carb-Fueled Macro Types have a tendency to have a high metabolism, so their body burns fat with such ease, they have never experienced a legitimate struggle to lose weight. On the other end of the spectrum, Fat-Fueled Macro Types find it very difficult to release excess fat. Then there are the those in between, the protein types, who are able to utilize fat for fuel effectively when dialed in with nutrition and training, but who can also retain fat readily when they aren't making mindful choices. Fat utilization can be optimized for each of the macro types by following the most appropriate cardiovascular training regime.

3. Your Carb Tolerance Level

Timing is everything when it comes to optimizing your training protocol by making sure it is compatible with your carb tolerance. Your carb tolerance will determine the best time of day to train as well as which types of cardio training you should perform. This is especially important because it can make a huge difference in the ability of those with lower carb tolerance to achieve their goals.

Resistance training actually increases carb tolerance because your body burns off stored glycogen during anaerobic exercise. Conversely, there are training protocols that could cause the body to experience fat gain and muscle loss, which we *do not* want. Manipulating the timing and content of your meals and workouts allows you to optimize the anabolic effects of the insulin hormone. For example, there are specific times of day, like right after a challenging resistance training session, that the body is more prepared to handle higher levels of insulin because your carb stores were just depleted. This means that the carbs you consume after your workout will not be stored as fat but rather will help build muscle. This is important knowledge because it can help you reap the benefits related to muscle growth, including increased carb tolerance.

Training Protocols by Macro Type

I have created five unique training protocols for each of the macro types. The Carb-Fueled Macro Types have the easiest time dropping fat but the biggest struggle to gain muscle. The Protein-Fueled Macro Types can lose fat when they apply themselves, but it's not as effortless as those who are carb-fueled. Protein-fueled individuals can experience faster muscle gains without as much effort compared to those who are carb-fueled. Fat-fueled individuals tend to struggle with fat loss the most but gain muscle with ease and don't need to lift as heavy to experience changes in muscle mass.

Understanding how the muscles work is the foundation of an effective strength-training routine. The human body has over 600 muscles, which consist of cardiac muscle (specific to the heart), smooth muscle (involuntary movements related to internal organs that support digestion, reproduction, and blood flow), and last but not least skeletal muscle (attached to your bones to support movement). In weight training, your focus is on developing your skeletal muscle, which accounts for roughly one-third of your body mass.

When it comes to weight training for fat loss, training programs are focused on splitting exercises among the six major muscle categories:

1. Chest
2. Back
3. Arms
4. Abdominals
5. Legs
6. Shoulders

If you are new to resistance training, most beginner-friendly workout plans tend to focus on a total body approach. I've found for fat loss and body sculpting, a split style of training works best. *Split training* means that instead of trying to hit every body part in each session, you divide your exercises into separate categories such as legs or core work or arms and perform the exercises for each category on different days.

Over the years, I have tried many ways to split up a workout routine during the week. Of all the training splits imaginable, my clients and I have achieved the best results with a **push/pull/legs training split**. This allows you to boost your training volume by hitting each of the muscle groups twice a week. Studies show that training volume has a more significant impact on muscle hypertrophy, which means that hitting the muscle groups twice a week will support *gains*.

With this approach, you will organize your training days into three main categories based on the nature of the movements. Bundling the movements into three main groups based on the exercise provides a logical structure to design a workout split at a training frequency of three to six times a week based on the following exercise groups: push, pull, and legs.

The push/pull/legs training approach is ideal for higher training frequency. Studies show you gain maximum muscle if you split your training to accommodate each major muscle group being trained twice a week as opposed to once a week. By training related muscle groups together in a single training session, my clients benefit from a natural overlap of movements. For example, on a push day, you are performing movements that involve a natural pushing motion like the bench press. However, when you perform the bench press movement, it also engages the shoulders and triceps. When you perform a shoulder press exercise like the seated dumbbell shoulder press, it also engages the upper chest muscles. It makes logical sense to combine synergistic movements together in the same training session.

PUSH EXERCISES

These types of exercises engage the muscles when you *push* weight away from the body. The primary muscles worked on a push day include the chest, triceps, and shoulders. I recommend that you choose five to ten exercises from the push list, and always start your push day with bench press as the first movement. If you are training at home and you don't have a bench, you can perform this movement with a push-up on the floor, on an ottoman, an ab ball, the edge of a couch, or even on a step platform. Keep in mind you can also replace any barbell movement with two dumbbells if you are training at home or at a gym with limited equipment.

The bench press is probably the most popular weight-lifting exercise of all time. It allows you to safely and effectively push maximum weight using only the upper body muscles. This is a compound movement that involves multiple joints and muscles. For this reason, you always want to order the exercises with bench press first so you don't prematurely fatigue the smaller muscles in the upper arm and shoulders with the other movements. This will enable you to maximize your training volume on your push days.

Push Exercise List
See page 298 for access to descriptions of the following exercises.

- Bench press
- Incline bench press
- Close-grip bench press
- Standing cable crossovers
- Skull crushers
- Tricep dips
- Military press
- Shoulder press
- Arnold press
- Push-ups
- Tricep push-downs
- Overhead extensions
- Chest flys
- Incline dumbbell flys
- Overhead presses
- Lateral raises
- Front raises

PULL EXERCISES

These movements activate muscle engagement when you pull weight closer to your body. The primary muscles worked on a pull day include all of the back muscles, biceps, and core. It is recommended to choose five to ten exercises from the pull list, and always start your pull day with the deadlift as the first movement. This compound movement is like the main course of your meal with the remaining movements serving as the veggies and sides. The objective of the deadlift on your pull day is to isolate the back; however, it also engages the core, legs, glutes, shoulders, and even the forearms. This should be your heaviest movement while utilizing good form and always using a spotter when training with heavy weight.

Pull Exercise List

See page 298 for access to descriptions of the following exercises.

- Deadlifts
- Lat pull-downs
- Barbell rows
- T-bar rows
- Cable rows
- Lateral raises
- Front raises
- Upright rows
- Seated low rows
- Face pulls
- Barbell curls
- Dumbbell curls
- Cable curls
- Hammer curls
- Preacher curls
- Shrugs
- Hyperextensions
- Good mornings

LEG EXERCISES

Training legs is best managed as a dedicated training day designed to target the lower body. The legs and glutes comprise the largest muscle groups and require a separate training session to support optimal recovery. I recommend you choose one or two exercises per leg muscle — quad-focused, hamstring-focused, glute-focused, and calf-focused — resulting in a total of four to eight exercises for the entire workout. Depending on your goal, start with either the barbell squat (more quad-focused) or barbell hip thrust (more glute-focused) as the first movement in your training session.

Leg Exercise List

See page 298 for access to descriptions of the following exercises.

- Barbell squats
- Barbell hip thrusts
- Deadlifts
- Romanian deadlifts
- Front squats
- Sumo squats
- Leg press

- Bulgarian split squats
- Barbell lunges
- Standing calf raises
- Leg curls
- Seated leg extensions
- Cable pull-through

CARDIO

A comprehensive training program would not be complete without the addition of cardio. The heart is also a muscle that needs to be worked just like the others to ensure overall health. Cardio can present a double-edged sword in that it's great for fat loss but too much can sacrifice lean muscle tissue. There are two types of cardio based on your desired heart rate: low-intensity steady state (LISS) and high-intensity interval training (HIIT).

Low-Intensity Steady State (LISS)

Think of steady-state cardio like driving your car on cruise control. You're moving but not applying pressure to the gas pedal. This type of cardio is where you elevate your heart rate to 40 to 70 percent of your maximum target heart rate. (This comes out to an average of 130 bpm for most healthy adults; however, you can determine your exact target heart rate using an online calculator.) Then you maintain it at a steady rate throughout your workout session. This means you sustain a steady pace like fast incline walking, hiking, jogging, running, or utilizing cross-training equipment like the elliptical machines. This type of training is highly aerobic since it relies on oxygen and, having burned through glucose, is fueled by stored body fat.

High-Intensity Interval Training (HIIT)

HIIT cardio alternates between intervals of high- and low-intensity exercise. Your training intervals should be performed at 80 to 95 percent of your maximum heart rate, and your recovery intervals should be 40 to 50 percent of your maximum heart rate. The intensity of this style of training makes it more challenging than LISS workouts, and you can burn more calories in a shorter timeframe. An example of this would be walking for 5 minutes on a treadmill to warm up, then moving into a period of high intensity such as 30 seconds of sprinting followed by a recovery period. The length of recovery period you need will depend on your fitness level. If you are a beginner, you may need 1 to 3 minutes to recover; if you are intermediate, you may need 60 to 90 seconds; if you are advanced, you'd utilize a 30 seconds on, 30 seconds off mode. You can set up these types of workouts with any high-intensity activity like a sprint, plyometric exercise, or advanced training movements like boxing.

Muscle Fibers and Macro Types

If you have ever wondered why some individuals seem to be able to run miles and miles without getting tired while others have a natural ability to go beast mode in the gym, the answer lies in muscle fiber composition. Your muscle fiber type impacts how your body utilizes energy, which means it has a direct connection to your macro type.

There are two main types of skeletal muscle fibers, commonly referred to as type I and type II.

TYPE I (SLOW-TWITCH) muscle fibers rely on oxygen as the fuel source (aerobic). They are also known as slow-twitch muscle fibers because they contract slowly and are great for endurance-oriented activities, like distance running, because they don't fatigue easily. If you took a biopsy of a slow-twitch muscle fiber, you would see that they are red, which means that they have a lot of blood flow. Slow-twitch muscle fibers are *not* fueled by carbs; they are fueled by oxygen because they utilize an aerobic pathway for energy. Fat is used for fuel via beta oxidation when it comes to slow-twitch muscle fibers. This is precisely why hard gainers are so naturally lean, because their body naturally utilizes fat for fuel more readily.

TYPE II (FAST-TWITCH) muscle fibers are called on for short bursts of power first by the body to energize your muscles. They provide the fastest contractions and are fueled by anaerobic respiration, using carbohydrates to generate energy. This means that energy is generated by a glycolytic pathway by utilizing carbohydrates to generate ATP (aka energy). There are two subtypes of fast-twitch muscle fibers.

TYPE IIA (INTERMEDIATE) muscle fibers rely on a hybrid of oxygen and carbs (aerobic + anaerobic). This combination allows for superior performance with respect to weight training and power-oriented movements that require a little more stamina. The beauty of these fibers is that they can handle a wide range of movements. They are a hybrid in the sense that they have characteristics of fast twitch in their ability to contract quickly, but they also have an aerobic capacity as well.

TYPE IIB (FAST-TWITCH) fibers don't use oxygen to generate energy. Instead, they use energy stored in the muscle cells in the form of sugar (carbs) that can be used for short bursts of movement. These fibers have the most power output but are also the most inefficient, resulting in a faster onset of fatigue.

Your body's muscle fiber composition influences how your body uses energy to fuel your workouts and helps determine the best workout regimen for you to use along with your custom nutrition plan. For example, a Carb-Fueled Macro Type has a higher concentration of aerobic muscle fibers that rely on fat for fuel, so if this is your macro type, you will have a natural tendency to be very lean without effort. If you want a more curvy or thick appearance, you will need to work harder to activate the fast-twitch muscle fibers that rely on carbs to add muscle.

• • •

Let's go deeper into the specific strategies for each macro type.

Training for Type 1: Carb-Fueled Macro Type

TRAINING

The Carb-Fueled Macro Type has the highest percentage of type I (slow-twitch) muscle fibers, so if this is you, you'll have the hardest time gaining muscle mass.

Your muscle fiber type is genetic, so if you are a naturally gifted distance runner who was born with two-thirds slow-twitch muscle fibers and only one-third fast-twitch, you can't create more fast-twitch muscle fibers, but you can make your fast-twitch muscle fibers *larger* by altering your training technique and nutrition.

The carb-fueled training program is best as a less-is-more approach. Less work is required to stimulate gains due to a lower tolerance for strength training. In order to build up the fast-twitch muscle fibers, you need to increase carb intake and lift heavier weight. It is recommended to train at 80 percent of your 1 rep max (1RM). You'll want to do between 3 and 5 sets, performing 4 to 8 reps per set, and taking 1 to 3 minutes rest between sets.

Be careful not to overdo it, as overtraining will lead to breaking down more muscle. Too much will impact your body's ability to rebuild torn muscle fibers. Remember, less is more: Less overall work will actually help stimulate gains. Focus your workouts on **fewer isolation moves** and *more* compound movement. This means that on your push days, focus on bench press and shoulder presses; on your pull days, do more deadlifts; and on your leg days, focus on squats.

CARDIO

Carb-Fueled Macro Types have the easiest time burning fat, thanks to those slow-twitch muscle fibers. They are able to access fat for fuel far easier than any macro type, which makes it extremely easy for them to stay lean year-round with minimal effort, on top of the fact that they also have a naturally high metabolism.

Because of this, if you are carb-fueled, your physique won't benefit from additional cardio. If you are the type of person who genuinely loves cardio, you can enjoy it, but know it will compete with your aesthetic gains and will require you to boost your caloric intake even higher to offset anything you burn. I suggest you do cardiovascular exercises three times a week for 20 to 30 minutes maximum, and keep these sessions at moderate intensity, within 60 to 70 percent of your maximum heart rate. Steady-state cardio is perfectly fine, especially if you are focused on adding lean muscle. Please resist the temptation to overtrain with respect to cardio. If you are specifically looking to add size to the lower half, biking is also a great form of cardio; just keep it under 30 minutes per session.

Since carb tolerance is highest for Carb-Fueled Macro Types, we don't need to rely on resistance training to induce a more carb-tolerant state. Thanks to your high metabolism, resistance training in the evening will be the ideal scenario because you'll have more "fuel in the tank." Plus, any high-protein post-workout meal consumed late in the evening will promote muscle building while you sleep. (The majority of muscle growth actually occurs while you sleep, not while you are training. When you don't get adequate rest, you literally compromise your body's ability to replenish depleted glycogen stores.)

It is *not* crucial to perform your cardio in the fasted state (aka first thing in the morning on an empty stomach). You can do your cardio at any point in the day that best suits your personal preference and schedule. The only caveat is if you are going to do your weights and cardio in the same session, do the weights first and cardio second. You want to have maximum levels of glucose accessible when lifting weights to support the heaviest, most powerful weight-training session possible.

Training for Type 2: Protein-Fueled Macro Type

TRAINING

Protein-Fueled Macro Types experience little to no difficulty adding lean muscle mass or dropping body fat, but it's easy for them to gain fat if their macros are off or they undertrain. A protein-fueled training program requires a foundation of weight training complemented with moderate cardio to support fat loss.

Those who do well with a protein-fueled approach tend to have more type IIa muscle fibers. The beauty of these fibers is that they can handle a wide range of movements, allowing them to excel at training to see results. This is why I intersperse higher-rep exercises in the protein-fueled training plan. This allows you to stimulate more muscle cells without having to load heavy weight for each movement, ultimately resulting in greater metabolically active mass, which is excellent for fat loss.

A hybrid plan of moderate to moderately heavy training works best at an intensity of 60 to 80 percent of your 1RM. Training should include 3 to 4 sets of 8 to 12 reps with about 60 seconds rest between sets.

CARDIO

Cardio is an important element to include in a training plan for Protein-Fueled Macro Types. This variable can make all the difference since it is just as easy for you to gain fat as it is to gain muscle. Consider yourself fortunate to fall under this category; your body is extremely responsive to cardiovascular training. If your goal is to lean out at the safest yet most effective rate, including cardio a minimum of three to five times a week for 30 to 45 minutes will be a useful component of your training. Do not exceed six or seven times a week with your cardiovascular training because it may begin to compete with your ability to gain muscle mass. I recommend that you split your cardio sessions between HIIT and LISS for best results.

It is also important to note that cardio is not 100 percent required for a Protein-Fueled Macro Type. I probably have your attention now! If your goal is to increase lean muscle and reduce body fat while you maintain your current body weight, you can cut cardio from your plan — but only as long as you are dialed in with respect to your total daily energy expenditure and your caloric intake. However, for those looking to get smaller overall and drop pounds, keep it in the mix.

WORKOUT TIMING

The Protein-Fueled Macro Type tends to have the most flexibility with respect to training timing. You don't necessarily need to wait until later in the day to weight train, but you shouldn't weight train on an empty stomach. It's ideal to eat at least 15 grams of carbs before weight training. This can be as simple as half a banana, a handful of blueberries, a slice of toast with jelly, or a rice cake. You want to have *some* glucose in your system to support the best possible weight-training session. Running on empty or running on fumes is suboptimal when it comes to resistance training. Of all the carbs you consume in a day, it's important to utilize them properly before a workout to make sure you have enough energy, and also be sure to consume at least 20 to 30 grams of carbs again after you train to ensure you properly replenish depleted glycogen stores.

Make sure that your post-workout meal is high in protein and carbs but low in fat. Fat will slow down the absorption of the protein and carbs into your muscle cells post-workout. Dietary fats are not bad, they just aren't ideal post-workout. Nailing the timing will be essential to sustain appetite control while following a protein-fueled program. You may find that as you train more to support fat loss, your appetite may increase as well. If this happens, make sure to stay mindful and don't eat "whatever" sounds appetizing in the moment. The key to resisting these urges is to ensure you are getting the right amount of protein to support slightly higher energy requirements for lean muscle tissue.

Training for Type 3: Protein-Fueled/ Low-Carb Macro Type

TRAINING

Protein-Fueled/Low-Carb Macro Types need to be very mindful with their training. Your training needs to focus on *healing*. The fact that you can't tolerate higher levels of carbs in your current state shouldn't be where you end up. Approach your training from a place of seeking to improve your carb tolerance level over time. This means that you will do the exact same resistance training as the Protein-Fueled Macro Type. Truth is, the only way to reverse conditions that cause low carb tolerance (such as thyroid issues, hormone imbalances, insulin resistance) is to push through them. Weight training is one of the only ways you can naturally boost your carb tolerance levels without medication.

Resistance training for the Protein-Fueled/Low-Carb Macro Type will activate the fast-twitch muscle fibers for short bursts of power first to energize your muscles. This means that your body will *need* to utilize carbs to create a glycolytic pathway to generate ATP (aka energy).

The first concern that comes up when going lower in carbs *and* still weight training is performance. My program is set up for healthy fat loss. While you may not be able to lift at your heaviest ever, you can still get a solid workout. It's important to remember that your training volume may not be as high as the Protein-Fueled Macro Type, but that is okay. Our objective is to boost your carb tolerance and support fat loss. You won't experience any significant hurdles to tone your muscles, but fat loss will be trickier.

The core of the protein-fueled/low-carb training program requires a foundation of weight training balanced by dialed-in cardio. Even though your carb tolerance is on the lower side, you still need to consume carbs for weight training to support building lean muscle mass. This means that you may need to go slightly higher in your carbs on training days and lower on nontraining days to ensure that your carb-driven activities are properly fueled. Because carb tolerance levels are elevated after weight training, it is possible to manipulate your body composition without entirely cutting out carbohydrates. This extra level of adjustment is not as important for those who have moderate or high carb tolerance; however, it plays an important role for those with lower carb tolerance and helps facilitate a faster rate of fat loss. Training with moderate to moderately heavy intensity works best at 60 to 80 percent of your 1RM. Be sure to do 3 to 4 sets with between 10 and 15 reps each and rest for 30 to 60 seconds between sets.

CARDIO

Cardio is going to be an important tactic for this macro type to help break down weeks, months, or even years of fat accumulation. Cardio will accelerate your progress, especially if you've been in a fat-loss plateau. It's key to ensure that your cardio sessions are a little on the longer side for optimum fat loss. It takes roughly 20 to 25 minutes for the body to burn through its stored glycogen, the first reserve of energy that fuels movement before switching over to stored body fat as a fuel source. For cardio to be worthwhile, it needs to tap your fat stores as a fuel source via aerobic respiration. Oxygen is the game-changer; it enables the release of stored energy for fuel.

The important takeaway here is that the first 20 to 25 minutes of cardio is great for burning calories, conditioning the heart, etc., but they don't "count" toward fat loss because those movements are fueled by carbs and not stored fat. I recommend a minimum of four LISS cardio sessions per week. While you can do HIIT if you are short on time, this can be a little too intense for some, especially if you fall on the end of the spectrum where your lowered carb tolerance is a result of a thyroid or metabolic issue or other hormonal fluctuations.

WORKOUT TIMING

Navigating low carb tolerance is all about strategic timing of how and when to utilize carbs. You now know that resistance training temporarily boosts carb tolerance. Another option to boost your progress is intermittent fasting. This works by giving the body specific windows of time for eating or fasting. This isn't about eating less; it's about eating in a way that minimizes insulin spikes. A typical intermittent fast is a 16:8, where you are fasting for 16 hours per day (8 of which you probably will be sleeping) and consuming all your calories in an 8-hour window while you're active and awake.

Each time you consume carbs, your body experiences a spike in insulin as the pancreas releases insulin to shuttle carbs out of the blood and into the cells. When this is happening, the pancreas is not able to release the fat-burning hormone glucagon. If over the course of your waking day, you eat numerous times from the moment you get up to the moment you go to bed, your pancreas is going to continually pump insulin into your bloodstream, so even if you've got your calories dialed in, you're not burning fat at the rate that you could. There is an opportunity to be more efficient by condensing your feeding window over the course of fewer hours, in this case over 8 hours. This gives the body a longer time for the pancreas to release the fat-burning hormone glucagon, thereby boosting fat loss.

The next thing to optimize is carb intake. The best time of day to include starchy carbs is after a weight-training session. Also be sure to do cardio *after* weight training if you are going to do them together in the same workout session. This optimizes fat loss because the body takes roughly 20 to 25 minutes to burn through glycogen before it switches over to utilizing fat for fuel. By doing weight lifting first, you can burn up stored carbs as your energy source during the weight-training sessions so that by the time you begin cardio, your body will be primed to rely entirely on fat as the fuel source during your cardio segment. If you are unable to schedule both workouts in the same session, get your cardio done first thing in the morning on an empty stomach and then weight train later in the day inside of the feeding window if you are pairing this with intermittent fasting.

Training for Type 4: Fat-Fueled Macro Type
TRAINING

Tackling body fat is the biggest training challenge for the Fat-Fueled Macro Types. If this is you, gaining muscle is extremely easy for you, but so is fat gain. Your progress will be slower compared to the other macro types, so please be patient and do not get discouraged. Stay the course and stay in your own lane. Be mindful to not compare yourself to others.

When it comes to training, Fat-Fueled Macro Types have the easiest time gaining muscle mass because they have the highest ratio of type IIb muscle fibers. This means they are great at short bursts of powerful movement. These muscle fibers are anaerobic in nature, which means that they do not rely on blood flow (which pulls from fat via beta oxidation). Type IIb fibers are larger and thicker and have a low oxidative capacity, which means they do not rely on fat for energy. Instead, they are more glycolytic in nature, where the energy is provided without the presence of oxygen by breaking down glucose for energy. Since fat is not readily used as an energy source for anaerobic training, and since fat loss is a primary aim while adding lean muscle, your resistance training needs to be more strategic.

These fibers have the most power output but are also the least efficient, resulting in a faster onset of fatigue. The good news is resistance training can turn the type IIb fibers into the type IIa kind, meaning you can train your body to become more energy efficient. Put another way, *you can train your body to become better at burning fat for fuel.*

For you, a higher training volume is best, with both higher reps and more sets for maximum results. Not only does this burn more calories, but it also boosts your metabolism and temporarily boosts carb tolerance post-workout. With higher reps and sets, it is ideal to train at an intensity of 60 percent of your 1RM or *less.* Keep in mind this doesn't mean to lift "light," it simply means to dial in the intensity to support hypertrophy. For best results, weight train four to six times a week with at least 4 sets of 12 to 15 reps or more. Keep rest time between sets to a maximum of 30 seconds. For an added challenge, instead of resting between sets, try adding plyometrics or supersetting.

CARDIO

Cardio is an absolute *must* for this macro type. Progress will be slow even with cardio, so if you want to hit a certain goal by a certain date, know that cardio will be an essential component of your success. If you are new to cardiovascular exercise, start out with a minimum of 5,000 steps a day for general health. For more moderate fat-loss goals, cardio sessions are recommended four to six times a week for 30 to 45 minutes per session. For *maximum* results, I recommend fasted steady-state cardio six times a week for 45 minutes, plus HIIT cardio sessions after weight training later in the day for 3 of those days. If you go for this higher-intensity plan, be sure to limit this style of cardio to no longer than 6 weeks at a time, and dial it back to moderate for at least a week or two before getting back into this style of intense training.

WORKOUT TIMING

The Fat-Fueled Macro Types tend to have the lowest carb tolerance with the greatest resistance to insulin. Resistance training makes a big difference in your ability to temporarily boost your carb tolerance after a workout. The Fat-Fueled Macro Type should aim for 10 grams of carbs pre-workout, followed by another 10 to 15 grams post-workout. This means consuming the majority of your carbs around your workout sessions. I suggest you separate your cardio and weight sessions when possible. This gives your body two windows of enhanced carb tolerance as opposed to just one. Translation: You can fit carbs into your day at two separate meals instead of only one.

Do fasted cardio in the morning, and weight train later in the afternoon. These two training sessions provide the body two separate opportunities to boost carb tolerance because your ability to replenish depleted muscle glycogen is higher post-workout, so you're less likely to store carbs as fat. If you are unable to split your cardio and weights for practical reasons, do your weights first, cardio second.

Training for Type 5: Fat-Fueled/ Low-Carb Macro Type

TRAINING

Thanks to your new eating plan, the Fat-Fueled/Low-Carb Macro Type is now energetically aligned to burn fat for fuel, making fat loss *substantially* easier. But when it comes to training, you may find that you tire faster and may not be able to lift as heavy as you typically do. The body needs to burn through carbs before using fat as fuel, so when your body is fueled by fats and depleted of carbs, that's when the magic happens and you are able to use fat for fuel. This is a game-changer, because your body can use stored body fat as fuel with ease. When you go very low in carbs, it changes the hormonal landscape of the body by boosting glucagon levels (the hormones that boost fat loss) and minimizes insulin levels in the body overall.

Resistance training is tough on this eating plan. You can build muscle without carbs, but your experience with lifting weights will not feel the same as it did if you were used to consuming higher levels of carbs. Your energy levels will be lower, and movements that tap into the fast-twitch muscle fibers will feel more challenging. You won't necessarily experience a new personal record with your weight training, but that does not mean that the workout won't be effective in changing your physique. Go into it with the expectation that you are going to do the best that you can, and if it means lifting lighter than you know you were once able to, this is perfectly okay. Keto is muscle-sparing; it won't break down your muscles for energy when the body is thriving off fat. While you *can* gain muscle definition on this nutrition approach, this is better suited for those with type 2 diabetes, insulin resistance, and hormonal challenges that present serious issues. This plan is also well suited for individuals who need to move away from dangerously high levels of body fat, seriously stubborn body fat, or if it aligns with your preferred eating style. Train four to six times a week, doing at least 4 sets of at least 15 repetitions per set. Keep rest times between sets brief, at a maximum of 30 seconds.

CARDIO

Now that fat loss is locked in because the body is using fat for fuel, employing cardio will take your results over the top. This is because you can tap into stored fat when performing aerobic exercise. If cardio is new to you and/or something you don't particularly care for, know that something even as simple as tracking your steps and daily movement can make a big difference. The key is to do *something*. Start by walking a minimum of 5,000 to 7,000 steps a day for general health, either outdoors or on a treadmill. If you are ready and able to give it a go, I recommend cardio four to six times per week for 45 minutes per session. For *maximum* results, I recommend fasted steady-state cardio six times per week for 45 minutes, plus HIIT cardio sessions after weight training later in the day on 3 of those days. If you go for this higher-intensity plan, be sure to only perform this style of cardio for up to 6 weeks at a time with a week or two of moderate cardio in between these higher-intensity bouts.

WORKOUT TIMING

The Fat-Fueled/Low-Carb Macro Type is the only one where it is okay to weight train in the fasted state. This is because, as a Fat-Fueled/Low-

Carb Macro Type, you are designed to use fat, not carbohydrates, as your fuel source. If you have excess body fat to lose, you can fuel your workout with stored fat in a fasted state. Those with the lowest carb tolerance levels function best with morning workouts because testosterone levels are highest at that time, and this also supports enhanced fat loss and allows you to tap into stored fat as energy. Similar to the Fat-Fueled Macro Type, you will do great with intermittent fasting by concentrating your meals into a shorter time frame, such as an 8-hour feeding window followed by a 16-hour fast. This will help minimize insulin spikes and support moving out of an insulin-resistant state. Also, dividing cardio and weights into two separate workouts is ideal because you will fatigue faster on this macro type's eating style.

Resistance training makes a big difference in your ability to temporarily boost your carb tolerance, especially after working out. As a Fat-Fueled/Low-Carb Macro Type, you don't need to eat any carbs pre-workout; however, make sure that you shun fats right after any workout. Instead, go with protein and small amounts of low-sugar carbs like a low- or no-carb protein shake with an ounce of berries. Fat consumption will slow down the absorption of the post-workout nutrients, so save it for later in the day. Make sure to optimize your carb intake post-workout.

TRAINING PLANS FOR EACH MACRO TYPE

Don't forget to access the training plans for your macro type online using this code. Using an Apple or Android smart phone, open the **Camera app.** Select the rear-facing camera and hold the device so that the QR code appears in the viewfinder.  Your device will recognize the QR code with a notification to take you to the web address. Exercise descriptions can be found here as well.

Epilogue: Macros for Life

I see people succeed with the macro type approach every day. They break through plateaus and obtain greater levels of health and performance than they ever thought possible. Some of them had tried almost every diet fad under the sun and were pleased to find a realistic, science-based approach that *works*. When I meet people who have hit or exceeded their goals, many of them are so blown away and excited, their positivity is contagious. This is a huge part of why I love what I do. That said, once you reach your body goals, what comes next?

At this point, your next step is to "reverse diet" into maintenance macros. On a reverse diet, you increase your caloric intake in small increments to adjust your body to a maintenance level of calories. You can calculate your maintenance level using the guidelines in Chapter 6 (page 145). The goal of a reverse diet is to add more calories from fat and carbohydrates over the course of at least four to eight weeks. Adding calories in small amounts boosts your metabolic capacity and minimizes the potential of regaining fat.

Reaching a goal you set for your physique is challenging, but maintaining that physique is the real test. While I recommend meal planning to help you stay on track, I know life sometimes gets in the way. This is where flexible dieting (see page 194) can be an effective means of managing your macronutrient requirements with more convenience and flexibility.

This approach is a spin-off of the macros approach known as IIFYM, or "if it fits your macros." Flexible dieting has grown in popularity in the last five to ten years, with more and more people interested in looking like fitness models, especially in the bodybuilding community. Professional physique competitors do not look "stage lean" all year. They only diet down to a "shredded" level when they'll be competing with the presentation and appearance of the physique for judges. This has led many untrained "coaches" or fitness "gurus" with no education in science or nutrition to perpetuate cookie-cutter nutrition protocols that are not based in science, and a lot of flawed practices have received wide acceptance as a result.

Let's be very clear: Your protein macros do not need to come from only chicken to be healthy. Your fat does not need to come from almonds and avocados alone. Your carbs do not need to come solely from sweet potatoes and asparagus. You are not sentenced to a life of restrictive eating! The macros approach provides science-based guidance on how to manage with precision the foods you enjoy eating. By knowing and recording the macronutrient breakdown of any food, you can have more flexibility with what you eat and still progress toward your goals or maintain your current physique. Flexible dieting requires that you track your macronutrients as you go, which you can do easily through a nutrition app, although some do find this tedious. When following an IIFYM approach, you set your macronutrient goals for the day, and as long as your macros add up in alignment, you can approach your day of eating and drinking however you please.

At its core, flexible dieting is being aware of what your food is made of and using that information to eat better. This means you can eat the foods you enjoy, even if they aren't healthy, so long as you track them as you go and adjust the rest of your foods accordingly. If you want a meal that is more on the unhealthy side, such as cookies and a slice of pizza, you can have it, provided you then adjust the remainder of your food intake to budget for it. This approach is the best of both worlds. It gives you freedom and flexibility but still provides the parameters you need to attain and maintain your ideal physique for years and decades to come.

References

1. Why Macro Types?

1. Thomas Longland et al., "Higher Compared with Lower Dietary Protein During an Energy Deficit Combined with Intense Exercise Promotes Greater Lean Mass Gain and Fat Mass Loss: A Randomized Trial," *The American Journal of Clinical Nutrition* 103, no. 3 (March 2016): 738–46, https://pubmed.ncbi.nlm.nih.gov/26817506/.

2. The Secret Code of Fat

1. Paul Cohen and Bruce M. Spiegelman, "Cell Biology of Fat Storage," *Molecular Biology of the Cell* 27, no. 16 (August 2016): 2523–27, https://www.ncbi.nlm.nih.gov/pmc/articles PMC4985254/.

2. Lisa Stehno-Bittel, "Intricacies of Fat," *Physical Therapy* 88, no. 11 (November 2008): 1265–78, https://academic.oup.com/ptj/article/88/11/1265/2858148.

3. Cynthia L. Ogden et al., "Prevalence of Overweight and Obesity in the United States, 1999–2004," *JAMA* 295, no. 13 (April 2006): 1549–55, https://pubmed.ncbi.nlm.nih .gov/16595758/.

4. "Tools and Calculators," *American Council on Exercise*, https://www.acefitness.org /education-and-resources/lifestyle/tools-calculators/percent-body-fat-calculator/.

5. V. Barrachina, "Leptin-Induced Decrease in Food Intake Is Not Associated with Changes in Gastric Emptying in Lean Mice," *American Journal of Physiology* 272, no. 3 (March 1997): 1007–11, https://journals.physiology.org/doi/abs/10.1152/ajpregu.1997.272.3 .r1007.

6. Sharon H. Chou et al., "Leptin Is an Effective Treatment for Hypothalamic Amenorrhea," *Proceedings of the National Academy of Sciences* 108, no. 16 (April 2011): 6585–90, https:// www.pnas.org/content/108/16/6585.

7. Beth Israel Deaconess Medical Center, "Leptin Restores Fertility, May Improve Bone Health in Lean Women; Treatment Could Help Athletes, Women with Eating Disorders," *ScienceDaily* (April 6, 2011), www.sciencedaily.com/releases/2011/04/110404151 343.htm.

8. B. H. Goodpaster et al., "Thigh Adipose Tissue Distribution Is Associated with Insulin Resistance in Obesity and in Type 2 Diabetes Mellitus," *The American Journal of Clinical Nutrition* 71, no. 4 (April 2000): 885–92, https://pubmed.ncbi.nlm.nih.gov/10731493/.

9. D. M. Muoio, "Revisiting the Connection between Intramyocellular Lipids and Insulin Resistance: A Long and Winding Road," *Diabetologia* 55 (October 2012): 2551–54, https://link.springer.com/article/10.1007/s00125-012-2597-y.

10. Naoki Akazawa et al., "Relationships between Intramuscular Fat, Muscle Strength and Gait Independence in Older Women: A Cross-Sectional Study," *Geriatrics Gerontology International* 17, no. 10 (October 2017): 1683–88, https://onlinelibrary.wiley.com/doi/abs/10.1111/ggi.12869.

11. Matthew J. Delmonico et al., "Longitudinal Study of Muscle Strength, Quality, and Adipose Tissue Infiltration," *American Journal of Clinical Nutrition* 90, no. 6 (December 2009): 1579–85, https://pubmed.ncbi.nlm.nih.gov/19864405/.

12. R. L. Marcus et al., "Skeletal Muscle Fat Infiltration: Impact of Age, Inactivity, and Exercise," *The Journal of Nutrition, Health, and Aging* 14, no. 5 (May 2010): 362–66, https://pubmed.ncbi.nlm.nih.gov/20424803/.

13. Marisa Coelho, Teresa Oliveira, and Ruben Fernandes, "Biochemistry of Adipose Tissue: An Endocrine Organ," *Archives of Medical Science* 9, no. 2 (April 2013): 191–200, https://www.ncbi.nlm.nih.gov/pmc/articles/PMC3648822/.

14. Beverly G. Reed and Bruce R. Carr, "The Normal Menstrual Cycle and the Control of Ovulation," *Endotext Online,* updated August 5, 2018, https://www.ncbi.nlm.nih.gov/pmc/articles/PMC3648822/.

15. Sunni L. Mumford et al., "Dietary Fat Intake and Reproductive Hormone Concentrations and Ovulation in Regularly Menstruating Women," *The American Journal of Clinical Nutrition* 103, no. 3 (March 2016): 868–77, https://www.ncbi.nlm.nih.gov/pmc/articles/PMC4763493/.

16. K. Shane Broughton et al., "High α-Linolenic Acid and Fish Oil Ingestion Promotes Ovulation to the Same Extent in Rats," *Nutrition Research* 30, no. 10 (October 2010): 731–38, https://pubmed.ncbi.nlm.nih.gov/21056289/.

17. D. S. Ludwig et al., "High Glycemic Index Foods, Overeating, and Obesity," *Pediatrics* 103, no. 3 (March 1999): E26, https://pubmed.ncbi.nlm.nih.gov/10049982/.

18. Sami Al-Katib et al., "Effects of Vitamin C on the Endometrial Thickness and Ovarian Hormones of Progesterone and Estrogen in Married and Unmarried Women," *American Journal of Research Communication* 1, no. 8 (August 2013): 24–38, https://www.researchgate.net/publication/261309731.

19. P. Vural et al., "Antioxidant Defence in Recurrent Abortion," *Clinica Chimica Acta; International Journal of Clinical Chemistry* 295, no. 1–2 (May 2000): 169–77, https://pubmed.ncbi.nlm.nih.gov/10767402/.

20. Sahana R. Joshi et al., "High Maternal Plasma Antioxidant Concentrations Associated with Preterm Delivery," *Annals of Nutrition and Metabolism* 53, no. 3–4 (2008): 276–82, https://pubmed.ncbi.nlm.nih.gov/19141991/.

21. Douglas C. Hall, "Nutritional Influences on Estrogen Metabolism," *Advanced Nutrition Publications, Inc.,* 2001, https://uniquenutritionsolutions.com/wp-content/uploads/2019/05/Estrogen-Metabolism-Nutrients.pdf.

22. Reini W. Bretveld et al., "Pesticide Exposure: The Hormonal Function of the Female Reproductive System Disrupted?" *Reproductive Biology and Endocrinology* 4, no. 30 (May 2006), https://www.ncbi.nlm.nih.gov/pmc/articles/PMC1524969/.

23. G. De Pergola, "The Adipose Tissue Metabolism: Role of Testosterone and Dehydroepiandrosterone," *International Journal of Obesity and Related Metabolic Disorders* (June 2000): S59–S63, https://pubmed.ncbi.nlm.nih.gov/10997611/.

24. Abdelouahid Tajar et al., "Characteristics of Secondary, Primary, and Compensated Hypogonadism in Aging Men: Evidence from the European Male Ageing Study," *The Journal of Clinical Endocrinology and Metabolism* 95, no. 4 (2010): 1810–18, https://pubmed.ncbi.nlm.nih.gov/20173018/.

3. How Macros Influence Fat Loss

1. Margriet A. B. Veldhorst et al., "Gluconeogenesis and Energy Expenditure after a High-Protein, Carbohydrate-Free Diet," *The American Journal of Clinical Nutrition* 09, no. 3 (September 2009): 519–26, https://pubmed.ncbi.nlm.nih.gov/19640952/.

2. Katherine D. Pett et al., "The Seven Countries Study," *European Heart Journal* 38, no. 42 (November 2017): 3119–21, https://academic.oup.com/eurheartj/article/38/42/3119/4600167.

3. Isabella D'Andrea Meira et al., "Ketogenic Diet and Epilepsy: What We Know So Far," *Frontiers in Neuroscience* 13, no. 5 (January 2019), https://www.ncbi.nlm.nih.gov/pmc/articles/PMC6361831/.

4. Discover Your Carb Tolerance

1. P. Kocelak et al., "Prevalence of Metabolic Syndrome and Insulin Resistance in Overweight and Obese Women According to the Different Diagnostic Criteria," *Minerva Endocrinologica* 37, no. 3 (September 2012): 247–54, https://pubmed.ncbi.nlm.nih.gov/22766891/.

2. L. Dye and J. E. Blundell, "Menstrual Cycle and Appetite Control: Implications for Weight Regulation," *Human Reproduction* 12, no. 6 (June 1997): 1142–51, https://academic.oup.com/humrep/article/12/6/1142/573355.

3. D. Macut et al., "Insulin and the Polycystic Ovary Syndrome," *Diabetes Research and Clinical Practice* 130 (August 2017):163–70, https://pubmed.ncbi.nlm.nih.gov/28646699/.

4. Lisa M. Caronia et al., "Abrupt Decrease in Serum Testosterone Levels after an Oral Glucose Load in Men: Implications for Screening for Hypogonadism," *Journal of Clinical Endocrinology* 78, no. 2 (February 2013): 291–96, https://pubmed.ncbi.nlm.nih.gov/22804876/.

5. Daniel M. Kelly and T. Hugh Jones, "Testosterone: A Metabolic Hormone in Health and Disease," *Journal of Endocrinology* 217, no. 3 (June 2013): R25-R45, https://joe.bioscientifica.com/view/journals/joe/217/3/R25.xml.

6. K. Fujita, N. Okabe, and T. Yao, "Immunological Studies on Crohn's Disease. II. Lack of Evidence for Humoral and Cellular Dysfunctions," *Journal of Clinical and Laboratory Immunology* 16, no. 3 (March 1985):155–61, https://pubmed.ncbi.nlm.nih.gov/3162025/.

7. E. Danforth Jr. et al., "Dietary-Induced Alterations in Thyroid Hormone Metabolism During Overnutrition," *Journal of Clinical Investigation* 64, no. 5 (November 1979): 1336–47, https://pubmed.ncbi.nlm.nih.gov/500814/.

8. S. W. Spaulding et al., "Effect of Caloric Restriction and Dietary Composition of Serum T3 and Reverse T3 in Man," *The Journal of Clinical Endocrinology and Metabolism* 42, no. 1 (January 1976): 197–200, https://pubmed.ncbi.nlm.nih.gov/1249190/.

9. Antonio Mancini et al., "Thyroid Hormones, Oxidative Stress, and Inflammation," *Mediators of Inflammation* (March 2016), https://www.ncbi.nlm.nih.gov/pmc/articles/PMC4802023/.

10. Gabriela Brenta, "Why Can't Insulin Resistance Be a Natural Consequence of Thyroid Dysfunction?" *Journal of Thyroid Research* 2011 (September 2011), https://www.hindawi.com/journals/jtr/2011/152850/.

11. George F. Longstreth and Brian E. Lacy, "Approach to the Adult with Dyspepsia," *UpToDate* website, updated December 9, 2019, https://www.uptodate.com/contents/approach-to-the-adult-with-dyspepsia/print.

12. K. Nakajima, "Low Serum Amylase and Obesity, Diabetes and Metabolic Syndrome: A Novel Interpretation," *World Journal of Diabetes* 7, no. 6 (March 2016): 112–21, https://www.ncbi.nlm.nih.gov/pmc/articles/PMC4807301/.

13. George H. Perry et al., "Diet and the Evolution of Amylase Gene Copy Number Variation," *Nature Genetics* 39, no. 10 (May 2008): 1256–60, https://www.ncbi.nlm.nih.gov/pmc/articles/PMC2377015/.

14. Abedelilah Arredouani et al., "Metabolomic Profile of Low-Copy Number Carriers at the Salivary α-Amylase Gene Suggests a Metabolic Shift Toward Lipid-Based Energy Production," *Diabetes* 65, no. 11 (November 2016): 3362–68, https://pubmed.ncbi.nlm.nih.gov/27436124/.

15. Peter Gibson and Susan Shepherd, "Evidence-Based Dietary Management of Functional Gastrointestinal Symptoms: The FODMAP Approach," *Journal of Gastroenterology and Hepatology* 25 (2010): 252–58, https://onlinelibrary.wiley.com/doi/full/10.1111/j.1440-1746.2009.06149.x.

16. Suma Magge and Anthony Lembo, "Low-FODMAP Diet for Treatment of Irritable Bowel Syndrome," *Gastroenterology & Hepatology* 8, 11 (2021): 739–45, https://www.ncbi.nlm.nih.gov/pmc/articles/PMC3966170/.

5. Identify Your Macro Type

1. Stuart M. Phillips, "Dietary Protein for Athletes: From Requirements to Metabolic Advantage," NRC Research Press online, 31 (2006): 647–53, http://www.insideoutsidespa.com/archive/phillips-dietary-protein-athletes.pdf.

2. Stuart M. Phillips, "Dietary Protein for Athletes," 647–54.

6. Setting Up Your Plan

1. *Body Mass Index, illustration*, November 4, 2016, Science History Images, https://www
    .alamy.com/body-mass-index-illustration-image353194322.html.

7. Eating for Each Macro Type and Sample Meal Plans

1. Alan Albert Aragon and Brad Jon Schoenfeld, "Nutrient Timing Revisited: Is There a
    Post-Exercise Anabolic Window?" *Journal of the International Society of Sports Nutrition* 10,
    no. 1 (January 2013): 5, https://pubmed.ncbi.nlm.nih.gov/23360586/.
2. Chris Poole et al., "The Role of Post-Exercise Nutrient Administration on Muscle Protein
    Synthesis and Glycogen Synthesis," *Journal of Sports Science & Medicine* 9, no. 3 (Septem-
    ber 2010): 354–63, https://pubmed.ncbi.nlm.nih.gov/24149627/.
3. Elsevier Health Sciences, "Increased Protein Consumption Linked to Feelings of Fullness:
    Detailed Meta-Analysis Indicates That People with Higher Protein Intake Feel More Full
    After Meals," *ScienceDaily* (March 3, 2016), www.sciencedaily.com/releases/2016/03
    /160303083809.htm.
4. Jaapna Dhillon et al., "The Effects of Increased Protein Intake on Fullness: A Meta-
    Analysis and Its Limitations," *Journal of the Academy of Nutrition and Dietetics* 116, no. 6
    (June 2016): 968–83, https://jandonline.org/article/S2212-2672(16)00042-3/fulltext.
5. Aragon, "Nutrient Timing Revisited."
6. Aragon, "Nutrient Timing Revisited."
7. Aragon, "Nutrient Timing Revisited."

General Index

Recipe Index

About the Author

Award-winning chemist and three-time champion fitness competitor, nutrition, and exercise expert Christine Hronec uses her background in serious science to develop her bestselling online body type programs. Since founding her company in 2013, Christine has personally helped over 35,000 women transform their bodies and switch to a body-positive self-image.

With over 25 million views on her YouTube channel, Christine has been a leader in the area of women's health since 2012. She's been featured in *Forbes, Huffington Post, Muscle & Fitness Hers,* and *Flex* magazine, and has appeared on *Extra,* Fox News, and CBS.

After more than a decade of experience as an engineer in research, development, and manufacturing, Christine leaped into entrepreneurship and founded a cGMP FDA–registered dietary supplement manufacturing facility. Once Christine crossed over into the world of sports nutrition, she combined her areas of expertise and founded Gauge Girl Training in 2013, now a multiple seven-figure international online meal planning and coaching service. In addition, Christine is the owner and founder of Gauge Life Nutrition, an all-natural dietary supplement brand established in 2019.

She's received awards from the American Chemical Society and was published in the American Institute of Chemical Engineers journal. Christine was part of the team that created *Time* magazine's Best Inventions of the Year for her work in the biotech field. She earned a bachelor's degree and also a master of science in chemical and biological engineering from Drexel University. Christine lives in Philadelphia, Pennsylvania, with her two pit bulls, Boss and Cash.